The Personal Development Book for Performers

Anthony King

Published by Faria Publishing Limited 2019

The Personal Development Book for Performers (First Edition)
© Anthony King, 2019

Edited by Debz Hobbs-Wyatt
Formatted by Polgarus Studio

All Rights Reserved. No part of this publication may be reproduced, stored in a retrieval system, or transmitted, in any form or in any means – by electronic, mechanical, photocopying, recording or otherwise – without prior written permission. The author and publisher gratefully acknowledge the permission granted to reproduce the copyright material in this book. Every effort has been made to trace copyright holders and to obtain their permission for the use of copyright material. The publisher apologises for any errors or omissions in the above list and would be grateful if notified of any corrections that should be incorporated in future reprints or editions of this book.

ISBN: 978-1-9160887-0-2 (print)
ISBN: 978-1-9160887-1-9 (eBook)

Disclaimer: This book is not intended to be a substitute for the medical advice of a licensed physician. The reader should consult with their doctor in any matters relating to his/her health. Before continuing reading this book it is recommended that you seek medical advice from your personal physician and follow their instructions only. The information contained within this book is strictly for informational purposes. If you wish to apply ideas contained in this book, you are taking full responsibility for your actions. The author has made every effort to ensure the accuracy of the information within this book was correct at the time of publication. The author does not assume and hereby disclaims any liability to any party for any loss, damage, or disruption caused by errors or omissions, whether such errors or omissions result from accident, negligence, or any other cause.

I dedicate this book to my dear friends,
Therese and Eivind

Contents

Author's Note vii

Preface 1

Part 1: Embracing the Creative Mind 9
Introduction 11
Self-perspective 17
Being Unique 22
Determining What's Possible and Impossible .. 27
Experts Get It Wrong 31
Follow Your Passion 38
Learning from Children 40
John's Story 50
Facing Your Fears 56
Living by Principle 61
Directing your Energy 76
The Psychology of Auditions 81
Expertise, Knowledge, Intensity, Respect 88
You Are Not Your Talent 91
A Star in the Middle of Nowhere? 95

Motivation and Drive 97
The Next Project 101
Don't Look Up, Don't Look Down 109

Part 2: Maintaining the Creative Mind 113
The Traffic Light System 115
The Life Timeline 140
The Internal Furnace of Fulfilment 145
Embracing New Things 166
Maintaining your Talent and Staying Well 168
How to Feel Great… have some Fun! 175
Conclusion: Acquiescing 180

Source Notes 183
Special Thanks 189
About the Author 191
Also by the Author 195

Author's Note

This book incorporates writing from my 2007 book *Dance Like the Stars*. I originally started writing that book as a teenager, already very experienced when it came to the arts. I had been performing and teaching professionally since the age of ten. However, since then I have gone on to teach tens of thousands of people to dance, including celebrities, sports stars, royalty and students; from all around the world. I have taken some of the elements from that book and added some new advice gathered from my experiences. This advice can be applied to creative people from any field – not just dancers or performers. I have removed most of the physical lessons and added additional information which will be released in a brand new book, separately focussing on the dance and performance. If I reference dance as an example, this can be interchanged with almost any field of the arts. I have noticed that the easiest thing for people to grasp is the physical aspects of most artistic expression. However, it makes no difference if you are rich or poor, powerful or weak, successful or unsuccessful; it's the psychological elements which motivate creative expression before the physical act. This book helps expressive people (especially the artist, leader or creative person) to excel in their given field. It looks at the simple things; things often not communicated in class, that are of utmost importance for creative expression.

Preface

I've often asked myself, when watching great artists perform, or admiring an amazing piece of art, music or architecture, what is it that makes it or them so special? What is it that differentiates the great from the rest? Do they have extraordinary ability or a connection to something greater that we will never know? Or is it a talent that can be learned? When we see a painting by Leonardo Da Vinci or hear an amazing piece of music by Beethoven, we see and hear something that leaves us awestruck, but where does the magic that we all recognise as genius actually come from? Could it be a particular age or demographic? It would seem that it's something more than learning a particular skill and practising a lot. The magic comes from the unique individual, the magic flows through them and it is they who are the key to unlocking that potential. They possess a particular mindset or belief and a unique way of looking at themselves and the world.

So before a musical note, a dance step or other creative expression is executed physically; it starts as a thought. Its manifestation is the interplay of mental, spiritual and physical processes. The physical execution is the last part of that chain and is often the easiest to replicate. The other parts take some understanding, effort and thought. For example, before executing a dance step it is vital that we understand **intention** in order to convey that step effectively for others to appreciate and admire.

Great artists or incredible singers who hit just the right note understand that this physical act is only part of the story. It needs passion, belief and understanding. Of course with training and repetition, it is possible to teach a person to move in a certain way or make a certain sound, but there will always be the 'exceptional few' who have that something extra… I like to call it the magic.

Schooling alone is not enough to master a craft. There is a big difference between a *true* dancer and someone who can *move their body*. Take for example the artist with longevity – who inspires and gives hope compared to someone who simply entertains and is soon forgotten. The difference is down to the artist: who they are, how they think and what they stand for.

An artist is always an artist.
A star is born a star.

They just need to find their calling. They need to understand themselves and then work hard to perfect their skill, whatever that may be. So before any of us start on that journey, it makes sense to think about **who** we are, **what** we stand for and **how** we can be the very best version of ourselves. After that, it's simply a case of letting the magic flow.

Dance Like the Stars Book 1 was originally a combination of articles and blog posts I'd written during the latter part of 2006. My primary aim was for the book to serve as an accompaniment for any artistic person – examining the psychological processes of physical expression. In addition exploring how to think like an artist and be unique. I see dancing as a physical expression of who we are; we can learn to become a better dancer or a better thinker, and I believe the same rules can be applied to all areas of our lives. I examine what I believe are the most important aspects of true artistic expression. Firstly in an attempt to understand *who* we are as individuals and not just artists; and secondly *how* to convey who we are to others through our creative expression – in my case through the physical movements of dance.

My primary aim, through this book is to encourage you to think about you and your own self-expression. For you to think about yourself and where you are going, and to encourage you **to trust in yourself and find your own uniqueness.**

The ancients, while navigating the high seas, used to look to the stars for guidance and direction. They would use the constellations to plot their course through the rough seas and stormy weather. The return of clear skies brought renewed hope and a clearer sense of direction. Likewise, the ancient Egyptians, who influenced the world we live in beyond measure, were highly proficient in computing the power of the planets, luminaries and constellations and the interactions between them. As they looked up, they believed, as did the Greeks and civilisations before them, that it was these heavenly bodies which had an effect upon the destinies of nations as well as individuals. Today, we still look to the 'stars' (in another form) for guidance, fashion tips, and inspiration. We place people in positions from which we adore them but are hasty to knock them off the very pedestals we put them on when we realise they are as fallible as ourselves. It's amazing how much power and influence the few wield over the masses. Pythagoras, the first 'philosopher' considered the stars to be bodies that encased souls, minds and spirits. It is quite clear that today as we look up to our own 'pop idols', the latest marketed talents and stars we should ask ourselves, are they really worthy of being emulated and adored? Should we not instead focus our energies on expressing *ourselves* to the best of our own abilities? Surely this is healthier than trying to emulate?

These are not only philosophical questions but are most relevant for the artists, dancers, actors, musicians and entertainers among us – the true artists that will at least strive to be the best that they can be. The artists that dig deeper. Those who understand it is harmony that is a prerequisite of beauty. That the beautiful poem, dance, song, piece of music or expression is only so when its parts are harmonious. The message is clear: you must search yourself to find that harmonious combination that will raise YOU up to the next level.

Some might ask, what has a philosophy and self-knowledge got to do with modern pop culture and practical advancement of their dancing, singing, acting, song writing and performing? I would say that anybody who asks that question is not ready for the answer, as it would be of no use to them. Instead of turning on the television or immersing oneself in temporary pop culture for inspiration and direction, would it not make sense at least to take a look at the real teachers who created the whole system that we live in today?

Budding musicians and serious songwriters might, for example, find out who exactly is credited with the discovery of the diatonic scale, the foundation of every piece of music that we listen to. Who was it that coined the word 'tone'? Who pondered upon the laws of consonance and dissonance for years? Who understood and explained them? They might discover who first understood and explained the amazing and often overwhelming effect of sound and music on the senses and our emotional state, i.e. music and its power to influence the mind and body. It is clear that even the modern greats like Madonna, Tina Turner or Paul McCartney would not have given you a blank stare if you talked about the details of their craft, because they understand the importance of knowledge – and if you want to be as great as them, then you should be looking in that direction too. They would know how the Druids used melody to heal, as they believed it soothed the physical body as well as the soul. How they also believed that the strings of their harps were tuned to the planets and why.

This, in turn, might be of interest to the curious actor or student of English and Drama. Especially one that has read *The Merchant of Venice*, for example. A different perspective on what the author actually meant when writing; "There's not the smallest orb which thou behold'st but in his motion like an angel sings". That same line of the Shakespearian play might become even more interesting to the theologian when we look toward the reference works and the words of 'Job' when he described a time "when the stars of the morning sang together". It is quite clear: art, music, philosophy, theology and culture are all linked and the true artist should learn from them all.

But don't forget: YOU are an individual. Follow your own path and your own dreams, of your own choosing. Always ask questions. Search for your own truth. Express yourself in as unique a way as possible. I'll leave you with the wisest words that I have ever heard from a teacher – the words of the first philosopher, Pythagoras: *"Know thyself."*

Anthony King

Part 1

Embracing the Creative Mind

The Psychology of Success

Introduction

My name is Anthony King; I'm a choreographer and a dance teacher. I've taught thousands of people from all over the world, from the absolute beginner to the professional dancer. I've learned that when it comes to artistic expression, it doesn't matter what demographic we fit into: race, age, size or ability, we all have the same fears and we all have the ability to overcome them.

A while back I was on the phone to a member of the world-renowned rock group Pink Floyd who have sold over 100 million albums. We were discussing some special choreography for a show; I'm going to tell you exactly what I told him. "If you really want to do it…we can do it, no problem, that's your choice, but you have to be in 100%. It's really nothing to do with me, it's up to you…but if you're serious then we can do it." He agreed, with a smile and a chuckle, and I hope you do too. The smile and chuckle bit is the most important.

Artistic expression is largely about fun in the first place. I'll be honest with you, and let you into a little secret, you probably don't need me to teach you anything at all. No, that wasn't a mistake. Artistic expression is not an external thing that you learn. There are some very special unique exceptions (medical for example), but generally, it's not something that needs to be taught or learned. Can I teach you a step, or a move, or a piece of choreography? Yes, of course I can, but to express yourself is to be yourself, the person that you really are inside. You are a creature of rhythm.

I am going to give a dance example but it can equally be applied to any type of artistic expression that you wish, as the same fears, motivations and drives apply.

Dancing well is a state of oneness, of being you and having fun. The most important thing to remember is to lose your inhibitions. When dancing, fear can be the big negative force that can imprison you and hold you back. Fear is not physical, it's a mental barrier we usually create ourselves. The bottom line is that dance is a mental expression of who and what we are and secondly, it is a physical expression and manifestation of how we feel. That's all well and good I hear you say, "I'll just imagine that I'm Fred Astaire, or Madonna, or Justin Timberlake and then I'll go out and dance like them...yeah right...you haven't seen me dance!" indeed, you would have a point! It's only the first logical step, but it is a first step that can't be missed or skipped.

There's no denying that results require a combination of actions and thoughts, along with practice and hard work – these are key. Different action equals a different result. The same action equals the same result. It's important though, that you think about each step separately before moving on. I'm talking about walking into a dance class and sneaking out, because you're scared or hiding at the back, or 'joke' dancing, where you pretend you don't care but really do, or staring through the window, wishing. Those days are over! As the scientist Albert Einstein said, "Insanity is doing the same thing over and over again and expecting different results." If you've always been too scared to apply yourself, or are always stuck behind those four or five amazing dancers at the front of the class, or didn't even have the courage to make it out of your bedroom or the moves in the living room: then let's start afresh. Think logically and truthfully, by taking a closer look at ourselves and our own thought processes. We will have a much better chance of getting positive results.

Now, some good news: however bad you think you are there is always somebody worse! I make this comment in jest, but it has indeed got an element of truth in it. The point is that we do not have the ability as humans to judge ourselves in an objective and fair way. So it doesn't matter how badly (or well for that matter) you may think you dance; you're probably not the best judge either way and you're probably a lot better than you are able to see or acknowledge. The French author Anais Nin put it this way: "We don't see things as they are. We see them as *we* are." In my opinion, she was right. I also think that this alone is the key to any expressive act and an expression of who you are. Remember that movement and dance are just self-expression to the beat of a drum.

Dance and movement are the physical expressions of a mental process. Let's take, an example, a young lawyer (let's call him Tom) that walks into a club with his friends. After a few drinks he decides that he is going to impress the ladies on the other side of the dance floor with some 'cool moves'. When he finally hits the dance floor, he feels that everybody is looking at him and decides to really go for it. He sees people smiling and decides to add a little bit more energy and spice it up with some comedy. Now he really has the girls' attention, in fact, they're almost in tears from all the laughter. So the young lawyer responds in turn with laughter and a cheeky smile, returning to his group of friends for the 'high fives'. Although this seems funny at the time it wasn't really the reaction that Tom was honestly looking for. Although the reaction to his performance was a joy to behold, it was a joy for everybody else – not him. Deep down, he really wanted to dance, look natural and be himself – not the court jester. He earns £100,000 a year, he's a success, a great lawyer, in fact, he's the best. Tom doesn't really appreciate the reaction he got. Even though tomorrow he'll be at work and he'll be the star! It's always the same story. He believes he could never be the relaxed dancer he wants to be.

Let's take a look at the problem

Straight off the bat we've already established that we're not accurate at judging ourselves in an objective way. So a message for anybody who thinks that they can't dance or don't have any rhythm: your premise is wrong and that's why you come to the incorrect conclusion that you don't have the ability. It is the thought process which is flawed NOT you or your ability. In a moment I'm going to show you why you're wrong if you think that you can't do something – but we need to start by looking at 'Self-perspective'.

Self-perspective

Self-perspective or 'self-perception' are how we see ourselves; or more importantly how we judge what we are able or not able to do or through assessment of our own behaviour. So:

Question

If I simply think that I can dance like Gene Kelly or the famous ballerina Alicia Alonso, does that mean that I can dance like them straight away?

Answer:

No, of course not! But that's not the question we should be asking.

Question:

If I have a negative self-perspective of myself or my abilities, can this fact impede my development and progress, regardless of my actual ability or the truth of the matter?

Answer:

Yes. Absolutely!

The main factor to consider is negative self-perspective and incorrect negative thinking. That is the killer that will prevent your progress in any field. False self-perspective is probably the biggest dream killer and the saddest one. If you're going to abandon or give up on an ambition then let it be based upon a **true** reflection of your ability and contributing factors, rather than a **lie** or an incorrectly held opinion of yourself. This will also include the opinion of others. We are all influenced by outside factors which we usually give merit and weight to undeservedly. Sometimes we take the word and opinions of others over and above our own.

Is it possible that **we alone** know what's good for us and our personal limitations?

YES.

Remember, things can change, and experts can be wrong too.

You alone are the best judge of your potential abilities

Why? Because only you know how far you are willing to go to do something or what kind of real commitment and sacrifice you're willing to give to attaining a goal. In fact, **you are the number one expert in the field of you**. You will always have the edge because only you know what's going on inside and the depth of your passion. The truth and the key to unlocking your true potential lie inside you alone.

We all know the difference between right and wrong or if something is really possible or not. The truth is instinctively hot wired into us. We don't need an expert or a teacher to enlighten us – although we might need a gentle reminder at times to reinforce the truth that we already know, deep down. My high school drama teacher, Mr Oades, reminded me one day after class: "Anthony, in the quiet times, when we look inside ourselves, we all know the truth."

Question:

- Can I really learn to dance?
- Can I run the London Marathon?
- Am I able to learn to play the piano?
- Is it possible to lose weight?
- Can I pass this exam?
- Can I get a degree?
- Can I achieve my dreams?
- Will I ever be in control of my own destiny?

Answer:

Only you know for sure. You are the number one expert in the field of you.

I know for sure that if you really chose to achieve any one of your goals you would succeed. If you made the ultimate conscious decision then you would find a way to overcome any barrier, or if you don't have the resources you might work a way around them or change the rules. Remember there is no fixed script or perfect map for achieving anything. Rewrite the rules, redefine boundaries as you go. You are free to do what you want and that is part of the fun. The creative genius Paul Arden is said to have put it this way, "You may have to beg, steal and borrow to get it done. But that's for you to work out how to do it." The bottom line… the parameters of your goal or dream should only be defined by its author…you.

We often allow others to define our goals and dreams and sometimes, even our lives. We came into this world as unique individuals and it's my opinion that there is no better feeling than being yourself and making your own decisions. It's one of the biggest tragedies to lose that individuality and uniqueness by letting it be moulded by the world around you, by allowing it to supersede your own opinions, thoughts and desires. Let's take a closer look at individuality and uniqueness.

"Most people are other people. Their thoughts are someone else's opinions, their lives a mimicry, their passions a quotation"

Oscar Wilde

Being Unique

I think that we all like to think of ourselves as unique people and we surely hope that we are, but what's the fact of the matter? What makes me different from the next person? The writer Alan Watts points out something very interesting (The Culture of Counter Culture by Alan Watts, CE Tuttle Company, 1998):

"We seldom realise, for example, that our most private thoughts and emotions are not actually our own. For we think in terms of languages and images which we did not invent, but which were given to us by our society. We copy emotional parents... society is our extended mind and body."

So, Alan Watts is saying that we copy our emotional responses from our parents. So is it possible that even that which we claim to be our inner thoughts and opinions didn't really originate from us? Now that's a thought! If they didn't originate uniquely from us and were possibly placed upon us, then what hope would we have for style, talent or anything else? Let's take a look at that though. We are trained beings; we do what our parents and teachers taught us, turning us into what we are today. We are bombarded daily with what we need to buy or think or consume, in order that we may be happy or popular. We are engulfed with the concepts of what our limitations are and our place in society. That we will never be like those amazing people up there in front of the bright lights and walking down the red carpets on TV or in the movies and magazines. We act as if those people are from another planet, different from the rest of us. That's just what is thrust upon us from the billboards and advertisements daily. We are being spoken to, literally all the time through advertising, TV and the media, parents and friends, colleagues etc.

Does the world influence you? Does it enhance your uniqueness, buying into somebody else's idea of beauty, success or morals, or does it detract from you?

Hmmm… so when I say to myself "I'll never be able to dance like that!" Am I being fair? Am I being honest or am I just repeating what I think to be correct because I'm not thinking *outside the box*, but inside the parameters set by other people (which are usually so limiting)? I would say that it's based on other people projecting onto you and you reflecting that back.

The key points to remember are that

- You are the number one expert.
- You define your own parameters.
- What's good for everybody else might not and probably isn't perfect for you or your set of unique talents and set of circumstances.

"We project our own unpleasant feelings onto someone else and blame them for having thoughts that we really have."

Put simply, this is somebody telling you, for example:

"You'll never go far"

Or

"That's a really competitive field. Do you really want to risk it?"

Or

"Are you really going to wear that dress?"

When somebody restricts you or tells you that you can't do something, or has such negative opinions of your chances, it is usually a reflection of them onto you, and should not be taken as fact. The idea was studied in depth by Sigmund Freud and is a 'defence mechanism in which the individual attributes to other people impulses and traits that he himself has but cannot accept. It is especially likely to occur when the person lacks insight into his own impulses and traits'.

That's an important point to take note of:

"Especially likely to occur when the person lacks insight into his own impulses and traits."

Again it's a case of, how can anybody, other than yourself, know what you're capable of, especially when they probably lack insight into themselves and their own ability? When somebody dismisses your chances, don't take it personally. Think about what they've said with the knowledge that you are the ultimate judge on what you can and will do.

Again, as long as you are being honest with yourself and are willing to put the work in, I'd trust your own instincts over critics. Hey, critics and experts have always made mistakes. As long as you know that and understand that people are very good at projecting their own fears and failures on to you, as well as their own lack of ambition, you're on track.

"Our doubts are traitors, And make us lose the good we oft might win, By fearing to attempt."

William Shakespeare

Determining What's Possible and Impossible

In 1970, political thinker Zbigniew Brzezinski wrote about our thoughts too. He points out that in the future, we won't even have to reason for ourselves, or that we won't know how to because the media will do it for us. The media will give us our definition of what's right and what's wrong (i.e. what is possible and impossible) and not only that, the moral choices and our (opposing) arguments. We will then regurgitate that, as our own point of view.

Of course, he was right, and of course, when is the media or anything out in the world going to give you the full picture about anything? I put it to you that you're going to have to determine for yourself what is possible and impossible for you. You should look for your own truth and uniquely have a point of view on it. As with your goals and ambitions from the mundane to the profound, if it's important enough to have an opinion on, then it's important enough to have all the facts and think about it for yourself. Decide what YOU think. Especially if it's something that you're going to base your life on. A decision taken in your youth might have an effect on the rest of your life and your level of happiness. You want to make the right ones as best as you can because you wouldn't want to regret something as big as that. The good news though, is that there is always hope. In the words of Jesse Jackson, "Keep hope alive!"

You can only act to your fullest potential with all of the facts (or as many as you can get). It's always good to know what the bottom line is, as you have the ability to trust your own instincts and to know what is right or wrong for you, (looks good or not). Personally, I'd rather have my own opinions than somebody else's forced on to me. I think that the word 'forced', although a strong word, is appropriate and accurate in this case. Why would you dream of letting somebody else tell you what to think or do anyway? As the adage goes: "Accept nothing as true that is not self-evident", and I would add "to me", not self-evident to somebody else. Why? Because the whole world can be wrong!

The world is flat, believe me, I'm an expert!

If you lived in the 7th century BC, then *SKY NEWS 7th Century BC edition* and school teacher, Mrs Maurice, as well as your best friend, McCarthy, Pastor Friar, Fox News panel expert (wooden 2×4 panel in those days) would be telling YOU that the earth was flat, and they'd swear on their eternal souls that it was! Unfortunately, they didn't have the luxury of disagreeing publicly in those days unless they wanted to have the luxury of being barbecued at the stake!

Question (Mother):

"Would you jump off a cliff if everybody else was doing it!?"

Answer (boy):

"Yes, mother, I would, because you'd be first in the queue taking me over with you."

The young boy might have a point. Just because you think that you can't dance or can't sing or can't do anything and the experts all agree, doesn't necessarily make it so. In fact, most people are followers and will not take a stand for what they believe in for their own good, so how can they know what's right for you, when they, in turn, take their definition of what's possible and impossible for them from somebody else?

"It is not worth an intelligent man's time to be in the majority. By definition, there are already enough people to do that."

G. H. Hardy

Experts Get It Wrong

Famous misconceptions may be easy to ridicule now, but it's interesting to note that some of the most foolish statements of all time were given as basic facts and YOU would have been put in the *looney bin* for stating otherwise. Now if some of the biggest conceptions and ideas in history can be wrong, could it be possible that your smaller negative ideas and conceptions about yourself and your actual potential might possibly be incorrect too? Let's take a closer look at a few examples…

The earth is flat…

It's a famous misconception that the people of the Middle Ages believed that the earth was flat…in actual fact, they didn't. It was determined a thousand years earlier, in the 6th Century BC, by Pythagoras the famous philosopher and mathematician, who advocated that the earth was a spherical shape. Even so, there was a point in time when people did indeed believe with all their hearts, that the earth was flat. Ptolemy, known as one of the greatest minds ever, advocated that the earth was the centre of the universe and that the sun revolved around the earth! We can look back and laugh, but it's important to note that these were views advocated by the experts, scientists and the greatest minds of the day. It is all too easy to make scientific and value judgements based upon what we take for granted today, on subjective ever-changing social norms, rather than look at the facts and decide on evidence (or reality) rather than bias and personal preconceptions. Usually misconceptions. Even the greatest of minds make mistakes and evidently big ones, but that's part of human nature. You can't always trust the expert! The real issue lies in challenging misconceptions, and our negative preconceptions of ourselves.

It has been said (unattributed):

"Many people have difficulty letting go of misconceptions because the false concepts may be deeply engrained in the mental map of an individual. Some people also don't like to be proven wrong and will continue clinging to a misconception in the face of evidence to the contrary. This is a known psychological phenomenon and is due to the lack of

will or inability to re-evaluate information in a more objective way."

We're now talking about the root of the problem: intellectual integrity. You want to succeed in any field or achieve any goal in life then you need to be intellectually honest, to move to your highest potential. We'll come back to that but first let's examine more classic expert advice and predictions from "The Seven Habits of Highly Effective Teens" (1998) by Sean Covey, "Six timeless marketing blunders" (1988) by William L. Shanklin, "The Not Terribly Good Book of Heroic Failures" by Stephen Pile (2012) and some of my own:

"You better get secretarial work or get married."

Emmeline Snively of the Blue Book Modelling Agency speaking to Marilyn Monroe in 1944.

"I would say that this does not belong to the art which I am in the habit of considering music."

Alexander Dmitryevich Ulybyshev, a review of Beethoven's Fifth Symphony.

"Who the hell wants to hear actors talk?"

H. M. Warner, co-founder of Warner Brothers, 1927.

"The horse is here to stay but the automobile is only a novelty – a fad."

The president of the Michigan Savings Bank advising Henry Ford's lawyer not to invest in the Ford Motor Co. 1903.

"We don't like their sound, and guitar music is on the way out."

Decca Records, when they rejected The Beatles, 1962.

"Television won't last because people will soon get tired of staring at a plywood box every night."

Darryl Zanuck, movie producer, 20th Century Fox, 1946.

"… good enough for our transatlantic friends … but unworthy of the attention of practical or scientific men."

BPC (UK Parliament), regarding the Edison light bulb, 1878.

"Sure-fire rubbish."

Lawrence Gilman's review of Gerorge Gershwins Porgy and Bess (New York Herald Tribune, 1935).

"If excessive smoking actually plays a role in the production of lung cancer, it seems to be a minor one."

W.C. Heuper, National Cancer Institute, 1954.

"The singer (Mick Jagger) will have to go; the BBC won't like him."

First Rolling Stones manager Eric Easton to his partner after watching them perform.

And finally, one of my favourites:

"It will be gone by June."

Variety, passing judgement on rock 'n' roll in 1955.

And all totally wrong!

Now, the good news is that all of these comments and opinions of the so-called experts, at the time, had absolutely no bearing on reality, the success of the product or the person. Imagine if they would have packed in and given up after listening to their foolish advice….no Beethoven, no Gershwin, no light bulb, no Beatles, no Mick Jagger, no television, no Monroe, no cars (as we know them)…imagine the face of the world today. All of these individuals had an additional piece of the puzzle, they could see the larger picture and could think outside the box, they just continued on their course…and it really is that simple…they just did it! They put the work in and succeeded in changing history and the world we live in forever. Doubt can be extremely destructive. William Shakespeare wrote: "Our doubts are traitors, and make us lose the good we oft might win, by fearing to attempt." He along with Monroe, Jagger and the others knew that doubt is overrated.

Taking a closer look … Lessons learned?

If we take a closer look at all of the comments, we notice a couple of important things. They were incorrect predictions – misconceptions – foolish comment. And more importantly: they had no bearing on reality or the outcome. Why? Because belief, perspective, opinion and viewpoint are variable factors. Humans are imperfect and inconstant. Truth is truth. Statement, belief, declaration, opinion have no bearing on fact – or truth. The problem lies with the statement, not with the ability to succeed or fail. It is only opinion. 'Belief is indeed NOT absolute, Truth is.' That's the flaw and that's why the experts get it wrong and why we shouldn't always trust our own temporary emotions or thoughts on a matter. Emotions change, as do feelings. We feel optimistic and happy one day; sad and upset the next. It's 'Belief', that people usually want, and it has nothing to do with truth.

Doubt and opinions are overrated

Belief can be a barrier to success. We should strive 'to know'. Knowledge doesn't involve opinion or belief, since opinion or belief has no effect on truth. 'Truth is'.

Follow Your Passion

If you've always dreamed of dancing, singing or expressing yourself creatively in another way, then start your journey. Any positive step will move you closer to finding your path; your truth.

Truth is not subjective or affected by foolish prediction or *misguided* expert opinion. When I say "Truth is", I mean that that is your actual chance of success when you take simple logical steps towards it. If you do this, if you keep focussed on your goal you will get there – regardless of fear or opinion. It is your behaviour that influences outcome, not opinion.

True Success: Intellectual integrity. Organisation. Planning. Implementing your plan precisely. Your opinions on your ability might be wrong… that's no bad thing…because we never know how far we can go…there are no restrictions, except the restrictions we place on ourselves. With accurate knowledge we are wise as we step towards a goal.

Without it, we are building a fantasy: an imagined reality and not a true one. Similarly if we base our actions on belief rather knowledge we are setting ourselves up to fail. The key is **logical planned action**. And once you set out on your path remember that it takes energy; productive energy. Don't waste that energy worrying about the consequences when you can simply set the goal and take simple positive action.

Direction is everything. With any ambition or dream, it's important to count the cost involved in advancing, without prejudice. Understand your mission, potential obstacles, have a plan for them, and know what direction you're going. Understand WHAT you are doing and WHY. It might take time and mental strength, but if you are willing to focus on your goals, are willing to be intellectually honest from the outset, make a logical plan and just take one step at a time, then you have a greater chance of success. And don't take short cuts. You'll have to work hard and you'll have to be mentally strong and focussed. If you can do those things, then you will understand the secret of success.

Learning from Children

"The only thing that interferes with my learning is my education"

Albert Einstein

I think we could learn a lot about ourselves by looking at the behaviour and attitude of children. The things that we all used to be. It's amazing how the magic qualities of childhood are literally bred out of us. Children are full of hope and are inherent dreamers. My opinion is pretty simple: we need to shut up and listen to our children and we might actually get somewhere and start enjoying life. Sir Ken Robinson, former board member of the National Ballet, recently delivered a speech on creativity and how the education system fails us. This is demonstrated in the many emails and conversations I have with people who say "they always wanted to dance", "always wanted to do this"; "my parents made me do this instead". A string of unrequited dreams…

So why didn't you do what you wanted to do?

Let's take a look:

- My parents didn't let me
- I didn't believe I could
- I wasn't trained
- I come from an academic family
- People thought that it was silly
- I didn't have the courage to follow my heart

To return to Oscar Wilde's earlier quote, he said "Most people are other people. Their thoughts are somebody else's opinions". I agree and this is applicable here. I discovered this at a very young age. Sadly so many never fulfil a dream that is their own. We shouldn't forget that as adults we are trained to censor and subdue ourselves, to wear social masks and to hide our emotions. The only time you usually really get the truth out of an adult is when they're drunk! Young children, on the other hand, don't know about these social rules. They are spontaneous. They are free to express without prejudice or fear of judgement. A child will show their feelings in an honest way. As adults –

we hide, we lie, we try not to offend, we deliberately deceive... honesty is replaced by something else when it could all be so much simpler.

So, can we change this?

One thing which intrigues me is how we feel as we get older. What have we learned? What would we do if we could start again? I think it would be pretty cool to work out the answer BEFORE we get old, wouldn't that would be great! I once spent a day in Birmingham teaching a dance workshop for school children and it was so refreshing. We sang *Willy Wonka* songs for fun. Then on the way back on the train, I sat near six naughty children causing mischief... so funny. I think that I was the only one laughing at their jokes. I always tell my best friends and I'm talking about the mature adults, "Let's go to a playground and play!" and they think I'm nuts. But am I? Where did the sense of fun go?

I have a lovely friend who lives in Slovenia and she has a playground in front of her house – when we got in after midnight one night we let our inhibitions go and had the best time, playing in the playground.

Childish, crazy, a waste of time? No, I'll tell you what's crazy.

On my way to catch my train to Euston from Birmingham, I was in a packed line on the underground walking to get the train. I can honestly say that I felt like a beast being herded to the slaughterhouse. It's been a while since I've been in the morning rush hour and I had to turn around and take it in and laugh out loud! Is this what it's all about? Go to school, to get trained so that I can join the cue of expressionless droids at Euston or London Bridge on my way to a job that I hate. All this to make money for somebody that I don't know, to go on holiday for two weeks, go partying on Friday night and start again on Monday. All this so that I can pay the bills and do it all again and again first thing every Monday morning. No thank you. I'll go play in the playground and sing 'Willy Wonka' songs if you don't mind!

In my experience I have learned something…your teachers, your parents and people in authority are generally not the foremost experts and authority on anything. They repeat what has been told to them: repeat, repeat, repeat! They will impose their failures and beliefs on you. They'll advise YOU to go and work as a slave as an accountant, doctor, lawyer, shop assistant, street cleaner, carpenter or plumber. PLUS tell you that that is 'good' and that is a success. Why? Because that's all they know! Nobody has told them that they can do whatever they want to. Now if that's what YOU enjoy then that is a good thing, but if you do it to satisfy your parents or because that's what everyone else thinks you should do -then you will have to live with it and you are *off your rocker*!

Now, of course, not all adults are full of it…just most. It doesn't take a rocket scientist to work it out…just take a look at the world around us, open a newspaper, turn on the news…what happened? Look at the way we treat our children! Look at the murders, wars and hate…I say that we should put an eight-year-old in charge of every country and we'd have a fairer, happier world for sure!

I know somebody, very close to me, who was sexually, physically and mentally abused. I've known them for a long time. This person's family loved to beat them, not smack, beat. It has affected them forever. They beat with belts, metal spoons, bamboo sticks, smashed spatulas on them; they even possessed a whip! How on earth can you ever abuse a child and be sane? It is clear that these people were just following their own vicious desires and were probably abused themselves… the point is that these people believed that what they were doing was right. They truly believed that they were doing good. Look at what our leaders are doing around the world, look at the homeless on the street. Adults are clueless; they actively encourage you to be like everybody else and NOT follow your dreams, and they will do it with a smile believing that they are right. People die every day for their religions and they kill every day for their beliefs. We should all take a look at our children and the way they think and behave. Wouldn't it be interesting if we were all childlike (not childish) and expressed ourselves the way we want? Real freedom. Mentally and physically, as opposed to the repression and unfulfilled dreams of most adults. No, no, not for me and it doesn't have to be that way for you!

Sean Covey's Book: The 7 Habits of Highly Effective Teens

I highly recommend Sean Covey's book to all, not just teenagers. It's great for anybody wanting to affect positive change in their life. His father wrote a book called The *7 habits of Highly Effective People*, which is also great. The principles are exactly the same in the younger version, but it's so much easier to read and has pictures to illustrate the points he makes. I find that good news is usually simple and doesn't have to be complicated. You'd be surprised at what you can achieve if you just make the most obvious changes and decide to become proactive and start to make positive decisions. If you're fed up of not being able to dance or not being able to do something that you really want to do, then only you can change that. Taking that first step is often the hardest… but to succeed you have to mean it. Think of all those New Year's resolutions that are broken before the end of January. Why? Because we don't want it enough. Because we self-doubt, listen to other people. STOP. Put yourself in a situation where you have no choice but to succeed, where failure is not an option.

Napoleon Hill told the story of a warrior who lived a long time ago; he had to go and fight a battle and had to make a decision that would ensure victory. He had to go and attack a massive mighty army, and his small force was greatly outnumbered. He packed the ships with supplies and loaded the soldiers onboard and set sail ready to attack. After he arrived on the shores and unpacked his equipment and men, he gave the order to set fire to the ships! Before the battle, he made an impassioned speech and said, "You see the boats going up in smoke. That means that we cannot leave these shores alive unless we win! We win – or we perish!" And they did indeed win; they had no choice or other course of action! If you want to start achieving your goals, once and for all, then you need to get that kind of burning desire, where you make a conscious decision …without the fear of failure, because you cannot accept the alternative.

The Great Chicago Fire in 1871 destroyed several square miles of downtown Chicago and was one of the biggest fires of the 19th century. The morning after the fire, the shop owners and merchants went to have a look at the smouldering remains of what used to be their factories and stores. They all met together and had a conference to decide what they should do. Should they attempt to salvage what they could from the ruins and rebuild? Or leave town and start over at a more promising part of the country. Well, in the end, they all concluded that they should cut their losses and leave Chicago, all except one. The one that remained stood up and pointed at what used to be his store and said,

"Gentlemen, on that very spot I will build the world's greatest store, no matter how many times it may burn down". Marshall Field's, of the world famous Marshall Field & Company, stuck to his word and propelled his department store to increased worldwide success after the tragedy. He had that fire inside him and there was no alternative in his mind, failure was not even an option.

Sometimes people get so sick and tired of failure or of not being able to do something and see everyone else around them doing it…that it can drive them down the path to success. This process sometimes takes a long time. It might take years and years for some to realise that they can't handle not implementing change and start taking some action because they just can't stand the alternative any longer. This is a pity, because if they can come to that realisation in later life, then they can do it earlier and enjoy the benefits for longer. It's just a mental decision. If you want it then go and get it. Or at the very least open your mouth and ask for it. You must at least try, what have you got to lose anyway?

I want to tell you a story about a dear friend of mine who was sick and tired of being sick and tired about one of his lifelong dreams. Before I do that, I just want you to take a look at a poem by Jessie B. Rittenhouse called *My Wage*. I urge you to google it. Do it now.

Don't you think that she sums it up really well, that universal truth, that the difference between you achieving a goal and not, is actually pretty small? Napoleon Hill put it this way, and makes the same point, "no more effort is required to aim high in life, to demand abundance and prosperity, than is required to accept misery and poverty". The key is to realise that at an early age, so you can enjoy the benefits now, instead of living in regret later, when you can't do anything about it. There is always hope and you can change today!

John's Story

John Dover, a successful businessman, owner of one of the top chains of bakeries in London, which he built from nothing – was fed up. Although he was a successful businessman who, on the surface looked like he had everything, there was just one thing that always bugged him. He was afraid of dancing and felt that he couldn't do it. This had a major impact on the quality of his social interactions and he hadn't danced for years. Whenever he went to weddings or found the courage to go into a club, he would just stand at the side and have a drink. The problem for John is that this had gone on for so long it was really getting to him. When he could bear it no longer, he reached the point where the unhappiness outweighed the fear of seeking help. Although in his mind, it was impossible for him to dance or be taught, he plucked up the courage to go to the dance school's website and make contact. This might have caused embarrassment; but for him it was a big step. And no more embarrassing than all those years of standing on the side-lines.

I asked him to tell me what he wanted me to do for him and what he wanted to get out of this, what were his aims? He was convinced there was no hope but there was a big wedding coming up, and it would be nice not to go straight to the bar when the music started. He went on to say that he was kind of large and shy as well. Interesting, I thought. The great thing is that he was totally honest and upfront from the beginning. He had nothing to lose and everything to gain. No ego and no expectations… We arranged to meet at the dance studios. John later went on to describe his fear when he entered the building and how it literally hit him and made him feel intimidated. Well as I saw him across the canteen above the studio, I thought to myself, "This guy looks great and very established." He explained how he felt and I told him not to worry. After we got started, I asked him to show me how he usually dances. He told me that he doesn't at all, and hasn't ever.

Interesting but not a barrier.

The curious thing is that because he had nothing to lose and everything to gain, he just listened and repeated and repeated (and repeated!) until he started to get it. After a few private lessons he said that he now had the courage to try and come to a public dance class. He came prepared, early and ready to go. He hid in the corner and tried his hardest, but he survived and met lots of like-minded people. It's a different world on the other side of the glass and everyone is in the same boat trying to learn. Now John started to come more and more regularly; within two to three months he had moved up to the front of the class and people were asking him how long he had been attending. John thought that this was unbelievable! He was just a baker who couldn't dance at all! But he was progressing because he took action; he took that first impossible step. But that's not the end of the story.

John came out for a drink with some friends, one of which was a casting director who was looking for one more male who could act, for a commercial. He said that John looked perfect for the job and could he come along to the casting? Now you have to remember that this is all a big joke to John…an MD of a big company, being asked to be in commercials…this was all too surreal! Well, within a few weeks John was on television in a music commercial. After that, he was contacted by one of the biggest dairy companies in the world who thought that he would make a perfect baker in their commercial too…big money and worldwide!

John's life had transformed in a matter of weeks and his confidence was soaring. He had learned to let go of his fear and to just relax. He had learned to dance and he had made lots of new friends along the way and now was on his way to becoming a star too! Wow! The transformation from that first email to now is shocking. But the most important thing in John's story is that he took the first fearful step and then he just proceeded to take more little steps. Just small steps, nothing immediately life changing or earth shattering and look at the positive transformation: unbelievable.

He is exactly the same person that wrote that first email, just with a different attitude and perspective.

Oh, and one more thing…the wedding!

Well, well… John travels off to his best friend's wedding and boy did he have a surprise lined up for his best friend! During the dancing, the announcement came over the loudspeakers to clear the dance floor… John was going to do a dance solo. He was going to perform! The music came on, he did it, the whole place erupted in applause and the deed was done. He had won, he had overcome another challenge that he thought was impossible and not only had he overcome it, but he also obliterated all self-doubt. But there's more… at the wedding he meets a girl who thinks that he's amazing and is so impressed by his amazing dancing skills. She moves over to London and they're now getting married! Now that's a great story. John is an amazing man and I am honoured to be part of somebody's dreams coming true.

Take the small step. You have nothing to lose. Take a look at the character Edmond Dantes in Alexandre Dumas' *The Count of Monte Cristo*. For the first couple of years of his imprisonment in the Château d'If, he sat banging his head against the solid rock wall doing nothing but turning to madness and then after a long period of time he realised something. He started scratching at the wall, and small fragments would fall off, admittedly they were almost invisible, but after a few hours, he had scraped off about a handful. He calculated that if he had done this for two years, instead of squandering his time, then he could have dug a passage two feet across and twenty feet deep. And realising this, the prisoner regretted not having devoted the long hours that had already passed, ever so slowly, to the task…however slow the work, how much would he have achieved in the six or so years that he had spent buried in this dungeon! The idea fired him with renewed enthusiasm. The message is clear: **the time you spend procrastinating – could be time doing!** Take hope from Edmond Dante (and John!). Edmond escaped the terrible dungeon of the Château d'If by slow, seemingly tedious fruitless digging through solid rock…but over time it worked for him and he achieved his goal. **All you need is time and a small amount of action toward your desired goal and you'll be on the right track.**

Facing Your Fears

YouTuber Rob Robinson737 wrote the following extremely insightful comment underneath Massive Attack's 'Angel' video, about three years ago:

"The video is about running away from your fears, the longer you run away from them the greater they become until you reach a point from where you can no longer run as if there is no land left for you to run on and there it is your greatest fears stood there right in front of you, and then you realise that these fears are just an illusion and that you confront them head-on and then they are frightened of you at the moment you start chasing them."

The video has almost 30,000,000 views and I encourage you to go and watch it. Massive Attack's 'Angel' is from their *Mezzanine* album, released in 1998. The English trip hop group didn't actually release their video at the time as told by **massiveattack.ie;**

"At the time of the single release of Angel, Massive Attack decided (for cited reasons as not capturing the mood of the song) to not use the already shot promo video for Angel (which had reputably cost £20,000 to shoot) to promote the single. For this reason, the video would remain unseen for over three years where it would finally see the light of day on the Eleven Promos DVD release."

The video really captures, visually, the tragedy of not facing our fears head-on. We have a choice and once we face them, we realise that we are only running away from ourselves anyway. This process is actually called 'exposure'. This exposure to your fears gradually can help you build a kind of resistance and lower anxiety until you can overcome said fear. Never be afraid of exposure. The great teacher Napoleon Hill said, "Fears are nothing more than a state of mind" and he was right. In fact, when you feel or can sense potential 'exposure' that is often the first place you should 'go' to grow and evolve. This is really expressed perfectly in 'Angel'. With regard to fear, I actually mean unfounded fear. Or the fear of fear.

For example, some fight or flight responses are perfectly reasonable and I am not talking about that kind of normal life-saving fear… I am talking about the different type of fear, the illegitimate one that is the fear of fear itself that we run away from often in our lives. That is what needs to be faced directly to advance creatively and it is expressed extremely well by Massive Attack.

Remember the words of the great Henry Ford:

"One of the greatest discoveries a man makes, one of his great surprises, is to find he can do what he was afraid he couldn't do."

Other tips

— If you need to seek professional help, absolutely do so!

— If you need some help from a trusted friend feel free to ask for it.

—Own your fears and face them head-on. They are part of your current personality.

—Write down your fears and evaluate the risk level and logically analyse the potential consequences of taking the risk.

— Reward yourself if you attempt to overcome it.

— If you fail, do not blame yourself. Keep working at it because practice makes perfect and every time you fail you gain experience and are one step closer to resolution.

Scientific reasons to face your fears head-on

Paul W. Frankland and Sheena A. Josselyn wrote an article in *Science* magazine called *Facing your Fears* (a PERSPECTIVE NEUROSCIENCE article – Science 15 Jun 2018: Vol. 360, Issue 6394, pp. 1186-1187 DOI: 10.1126/science.aau0035) and they stated something very interesting;

"… treating no-longer-threatening situations as dangerous may be maladaptive and lead to anxiety disorders, including phobias and post-traumatic stress disorder. Central to many forms of therapy designed to tackle these anxiety disorders is the idea that to overcome fear, one needs to face it."

Maladaptive is defined as "not adjusting adequately or appropriately to the environment or situation". So this means that scientifically speaking, facing your fears is the healthy thing to do because if you don't it can lead to, as they clearly state, "anxiety disorders, including phobias and post-traumatic stress disorder". So, not only is it the logical thing to do, but it is also healthy for you… and most often, easier than you suspect.

Your creative prime is on the other side of your fear

This is why an artist has to constantly push their internal and external boundaries to expand creatively. This is all part of the creative journey and nothing to worry about because it's a never-ending expansion. Every artist will have some kind of fear before they pass it and extend outside of their comfort zone. Once they reach their destination, it begins again… that's just the way it is! It's the same for us all. Once you understand this then the fear of fear fades. That means that your greatest painting, greatest composition or greatest work is just one step outside of your comfort zone, through the fear zone… it's right there if you want it!

Living by Principle

Principle
noun
1. a fundamental truth or proposition that serves as the foundation for a system of belief or behaviour or for a chain of reasoning. "the basic principles of justice"…
synonyms: truth, proposition, concept, idea, theory, postulate…
2. a general scientific theorem or law that has numerous special applications across a wide field.

Philosophically speaking there are actually arguments *against* living and sticking to rigid principles. The argument is essentially that we should be fluid and flexible in the face of ever-changing circumstances. However, I am going to look at this idea *practically* speaking, rather than philosophically speaking. If we do this, then it comes down to one thing, in my opinion:

Optimising your creative artistic energy, efficiency and mental well-being is the main reason you should stick by your own principles.

You can't live a productive life against your own principles and nature anyway, so what's the point in even trying? There are numerous examples from daily life but I will give a small one. We have all experienced being around somebody that we don't like or even hate but are forced to be polite to, maybe at dinner or a social gathering. It's tiring and fatiguing to have to act, against your own nature and pretend to like the person. Afterwards, we notice that we may feel, uncomfortable, tired and uneasy (I previously mentioned that children usually don't do this and that it is learned). This is because our true self rejects the idea that we should pretend and act against our own beliefs and nature, and so it rebels against ourselves. In a way, we are disgusted at our own weakness and dishonesty to just *go along to get along*. This means that it is your own consciousness which creates that uncomfortable feeling which is a consequence of doing something which is not good for you or against your better judgement. That feeling can also be described as 'pressure' or 'headache'… when you keep something in but would really like to scream about it. If you engage in this regularly so that the habit becomes a lifestyle (maybe at work in your office, around colleagues you actually dislike but pretend to like ... how fatiguing!) you will see that it erodes who you are and will cause you pain, discomfort and is not conducive to your well-being or your artistic creativity. The irony is, is that the mild 'discomfort' at expressing how you actually feel and living authentically is much less painful, less tiring and less stressful than masking those feeling with pretence.

Either way, it makes no difference because eventually, the consequences will manifest themselves. The question is this though: why do something which is uncomfortable, makes you unhappy, is against your true self and is of no actual benefit to your life? Why not be free and say how you really feel? Why not live your life aligned with your true self?

Obviously, at root, *fear* is the answer.

However, I say that it's crazy because it's inefficient and not conducive to your own success. That is reason alone to reduce the 'fake' act and align yourself publicly with your private real thoughts and feelings on any matter or interaction. This freedom will make you more productive, efficient and happy. It is an action that very few people take, unfortunately for them.

Other good reasons to live honestly by your principles

It's not only constructive to your own aims to live your life by principle, it's also the right thing to do morally and logistically. I will give you an example.

Question:

Do you think that people who choose not to live by principle and integrity are good to be around?

Answer:

The people that lack principle are also direct threats to you and your creative aims. People that lack principle are quick to sabotage your desires and aims and don't often help advance your goals. Another reason to live by principle is that it projects strength. People will see that you speak the truth, stand by your convictions and aren't afraid to express how you feel. This is of much intrinsic value and elicits trust. Finally, one of the most important reasons to live by strong principle is that it is the right thing to do. Sometimes, you don't need a reason other than that. I will give you an example where I faced a life-changing choice, which was based on a matter of principle.

Standing up for the victims and alleged victims of child abuse

I have been linked to Michael Jackson professionally since I was a child. I first started off at around the age of ten years old modelling Michael Jackson's original 'Herb Ritts' costume and also wearing Michael Jackson's original 'Jackson 5' jacket, at Sony Studios promoting Michael Jackson's *HIStory* album. I actually modelled Michael Jackson's black 'Pepsi' commercial jacket, starring James Safechuck, in 1993, when I was even younger. Since that day, I have been involved with almost every official Michael Jackson album or project, one way or another.

Michael Jackson's Official website featured me and my 'Anthony King's Michael Jackson Dance Class' on Monday 15th August 2005. It was the top news story on his website… in fact it was entitled 'Breaking News'. It was around the time after Michael's child abuse trial. It has been reported on BBC Breakfast and was seen worldwide. I was always a positive story for Michael Jackson's P.R team and record company, which is why I have been interviewed and featured as a Michael Jackson 'expert' for Sky News, BBC News, ITV, Channel 4, ITN, CNN, Channel 5 and too many channels and the publications to mention, including even the *Financial Times*. I have filmed a 'How to Moonwalk' lesson which was featured on YouTube. As in, actually featured by YouTube, on their homepage… not once, but twice. It has over 35 million views.

I have taught tens of thousands of people to dance like Michael Jackson, all around the world. I have performed to hundreds of thousands of people, all around the world. I have taught some of the biggest celebrities in the world how to dance like Michael Jackson. I've taught members of two Royal families, I have taught sports stars and people that I watch on television from the England football team, celebrities from literally the biggest movies of all time to Miss World. I have forgotten how many amazing people I have taught to dance like Michael

Jackson. Billionaires… their children, their families. I've also held team building classes and taught employees from the world's biggest companies and you might have heard of a few: Google, Twitter, Lego, American Express, Red Bull, Anglo American, PwC, King (creators of Candy Crush), Cisco Systems, Proctor & Gamble, Metro Newspaper group… even our friends at the HM Treasury Department!

I have produced and starred in three *Learn to Dance Like Michael Jackson* DVDs and have written six 'Michael Jackson' books:

Michael Jackson and Classical Music
Anthony King's Guide to Michael Jackson's Dangerous Tour
Anthony King's Guide to Michael Jackson's HIStory Tour
Michael Jackson Fact Check by Anthony King

… and two unpublished books, that were almost completed that were to come out in 2019. Two of the above books are around 600 pages long. I wrote them to get this accumulated knowledge out of my head. I have even 'fact checked' the National Portrait Galleries official book and around 100 of the 'top' Michael Jackson books and their lies and untruths. I then presented those findings in my book *Michael Jackson Fact Check*.

Doing the right thing is always the best thing to do creatively

I believed the victims in Dan Reed's 2019 documentary *Leaving Neverland* and I believed them before the documentary aired. I had always been concerned by Michael Jackson's inappropriate behaviour with children and it came to a point where it was preposterous, after decades of abuse allegations by so many children and their families, to believe that Michael Jackson wasn't a child abuser. I then had a decision to make. In fact, it was a very easy decision. I was to launch two Michael Jackson books and decided that I would state my position publicly before they were published. I wanted to live authentically and support the victims who I believed. Two weeks before the airing of *Leaving Neverland* I put out this public statement:

"My thoughts on 'Leaving Neverland'…

Michael Jackson was probably one of the greatest performers ever and we collectively loved him and in many cases dedicated our lives to his art. However, Michael Jackson's (admitted) behaviour with children was unquestionably inappropriate. Adults sleeping or being in a bed with children is unacceptable. It must be condemned and never portrayed as acceptable and normalised. Children need to be protected from abuse and never be put in ambiguous environments, as our number one priority. The people attacking victims and alleged victims of child abuse are part of the problem. I won't immediately be watching 'Leaving Neverland' but people must be allowed to make up their own minds without fear of being attacked.

#michaeljackson
#leavingneverland"

I was attacked. Immediately. I received over 1000 threats including death threats, from Michael Jackson 'fans' and 'friends'. I was interviewed by Jamie Lee Curtis Taete of Vice News who wrote about the threats in his article, "Michael Jackson Stans React to 'Leaving Neverland' with Bus Ads and Death Threats – in the lead up to the premiere of the documentary this weekend, Jackson fans were ramping up their attempts to discredit the film".

He described the reaction to my initial statement;

"As a dance instructor and Jackson expert, Anthony King has written multiple books about the singer, led Michael Jackson-themed team building workshops, taught Michael Jackson dance classes, and released several Michael Jackson dance workout DVDs. A YouTube video of him teaching the moonwalk has been viewed over 35 million times. But now, he says, he's finished. "As far as I'm concerned, it's over," he told me in a phone interview. "I've removed Michael Jackson's name [from] my Twitter bios, my Instagram, and I'm working on literally doing a Pharaoh Akhenaten—they removed the guy's name from ancient Egypt, every statue, and I'm doing it."

Leaving Neverland's impending release prompted King to post a series of tweets in which he said that, regardless of whether or not Jackson ever molested any children, everyone should be able to agree that it's unacceptable for an adult to share a bed with a child in the way the singer allegedly did. He also wrote that it's wrong to attack "victims and alleged victims of child abuse."

The tweets were not well received.

In the days since posting, King has been sent thousands of messages from Jackson fans. Most just tweeted the reasons they believe Jackson is innocent. But some went further. Several people implied that King was projecting his own pedophilic sexual fantasies on to Jackson. Others called him "inhuman" and "scum" and "a dumbass bitch." One guy commented on his Facebook, telling him that he'd just burned his book. Some told him they hoped he would one day be falsely accused of child abuse, or have his own children be sexually abused. "U are so effin lucky u don't live closer to me," wrote one fan in a Facebook message. "I swear to almighty God up above I wud tear you from limb to limb" (sic).

This backlash, coupled with the new attention on the accusations against Jackson, made King decide to completely sever ties with the singer and his music. He said he'll be cancelling all of his upcoming Michael Jackson dance classes, and doesn't plan to start any new Jackson-related projects. "This is my whole life…" he said. "I just feel like it is the right thing… When the dust settles, I wanna be on the right side."

Being silent when you know you should speak will kill your creativity

Even though I had worked for years on building my Michael Jackson career and invested in shows and directly invested eighteen months in writing books on Michael Jackson, I knew that it was my duty to end my association with him and cancel everything. I was alone in the "Michael Jackson" world, as I was the only one who spoke out. Not a single individual linked to Michael Jackson defended the victims honour, publicly. They victim blamed, called them liars, defended child abuse or remained silent. I watched the victim shaming, attacks and also watched all of the enablers and people who had a duty of care towards the children around Michael Jackson for decades sit silently while the victims were publicly crucified. Many of them messaged me privately but were too fearful to speak out publicly. For me, to live with that shame would be much more painful than to lose my life's works. To the contrary, this was such a privilege to dissociate because I believe that when you live by principle you will be free to really start achieving and reaching your true potential. I then released a second statement to destroy the association with Michael Jackson and his fans, beyond repair:

"When you abuse a child you are no longer a human being, in my eyes. When you stand by and let a child

be abused on your watch, you are no longer a normal human being, in my eyes. When you are silent and an enabler, apologist and accomplice, you are no longer a normal human being, in my eyes. I condemn him and his whole community and supporters and followers. He and they offend me. They disgust me. Now… let's get down to business!

— My "Learn to dance like Michael Jackson" DVDs are pulled. Cancelled and removed.
— My "Michael Jackson" dance lesson downloads are pulled. Cancelled and removed.
— My "Michael Jackson Dance Class" is permanently cancelled.
— I will never teach another person to dance like Michael Jackson in my life.
— I will never dance like Michael Jackson again in my life.
— I will never listen to a Michael Jackson song in my life.
— I will never perform a Michael Jackson show in my life.
— Two of my Michael Jackson books are cancelled. All the videos that I recorded in many countries around the world related to Michael Jackson are now cancelled.
— My books have already been edited to include

condemnations of Michael Jackson.
— Four of my books will remain published because they are part of MY history but they will not be promoted or advertised in any way. They are just "Music history" books now.
— All of my biographies and websites are currently being amended as we speak to remove Michael Jackson and condemn him.
— If you support Michael Jackson or listen to him, I will consider you a child abuse enabler and supporter. So don't bring that anywhere near me and stay very far away from me. I can't be clearer than that.

#mutemichaeljackson is not enough. To mute somebody, they need to exist. If you abuse children, you do not exist and should be removed from society along with your enablers, supporters and apologists".

Don't live in fear, stand by your principles ... you decide what they are

Stick by your principles and you will elevate, creatively higher than you ever thought. I am speaking not just creatively but I am also speaking literally in every area of your life. You may experience some resistance but in the end, when you look back, you will see that you did the right thing for your soul, for your creativity and for your life and for others. If you choose to 'sell out', or 'live a lie' or be silent when you know you should speak, you are only sabotaging and killing your own soul and creativity. Nothing is worth that… and I mean nothing because it is not an optimum way of living. You will eventually reject it anyway, so you might as well do it at the soonest possible opportunity. An artist and creative person needs to be free and without those self-imposed mental burdens. Alleviating them will open a brand new positive chapter. One where you can be free to create and express without fear. What are your principles? Only you know when you look inside, but once you do look honestly inwards, your conscience and intuition will tell you pretty quickly… don't fight it. It's futile anyway.

Directing your Energy

It's very important to evaluate yourself and your energy consumption. I am not talking about your calorie intake here. This is going to be a short chapter but an extremely important one. If you don't eat your full quota of calories then you will be running a calorie deficit. This means that you will lose weight. It also means that you will feel tired, run down and not completely efficient. The same goes for your social interactions. In fact, it goes for every single interaction of your life and not just the people you know. You can exert energy in people and situations which are a complete waste of your time and life force. Considering that you have limited time on earth and also have limited energy, it's important that you focus that energy into goals and people that are useful. It's also important that it is directed in people and situations that are healthy for you. Including where you consciously want it. It's very easy to waste your energy and actually have it 'stolen'. We all are aware of the term 'energy vampires' and we are told that at least one in twenty people are psychopaths. So that means that 5% of the people that you meet will be inclined to 'suck you dry', energetically and emotionally speaking. However, I suspect that the number is much higher than that. So it's important to be aware and to only direct your precious energy where you want it to go.

It is very possible that when you analyse the interactions in your own life, you may realise that your 'friends' are actually harmful to you and completely non aligned with your goals, philosophy and energy. They may hinder and harm you more than help. Ironically, this determination can sometimes be clouded due to our emotional connection to the said people. This means that the people closest to you are the hardest to accurately 'judge' since we are often blinded by an emotional attachment and rationalise unhealthy behaviour of those close to us. In other words, it's important that you look at your relationships and make a determination as to whether the energy you put into them is appreciated or a hindrance to you. The people that you consider close to you, like your friends and colleagues, are often the worst people for you to be around. Have you heard the saying

'Keep your friends close and your enemies closer'? Some say it's from the Chinese military strategist Sun-Tzu and I seem to remember reading it in Machiavelli's *The Prince* and later repeated by *The Godfather's* Michael Corleone. However, the message is clear; it's not the people 'over there' that destroy you. It's the people close to you. That means friends and acquaintances. Bear this in mind and guard your inner space and only allow it to be occupied by trustworthy deserving people. The way to determine this is to analyse your interactions and relationships logically. It's better to do this sooner rather than later because you may find that you realise that the people around you are holding you back, a little bit too late!

Another thing to look out for is that if somebody is sitting in a dark room for a long period of time and you walk in and turn on a bright light and illuminate the whole room, then it will not be a comfortable experience for the occupant. It will probably hurt their eyes and they will usually run to turn off the light and shut it down. This example can also be taken literally. Sometimes your light will not be appreciated by those around you and will be shut down with negativity. Ironically, because we don't have something to judge against, sometimes we don't realise what's happening until we are old or it's too late to take evasive action. These are very important principles. You want to save your energy for those moments in life when you need it. There will be moments where you need to psych yourself up and give all you have to give to achieve a goal and to push yourself beyond your usual limits. You will need the energy to do so and if you have wasted it and depleted it on energy vampires and interactions that are draining, you will not succeed as you should. One final thing on this subject: advice. Never take advice from your friends unless you trust them with your future and your life. Never. Why? The reason is that you will always do what YOU want to do, regardless of what friends tell you. Even if you make the wrong decision you will hold it against your friend if the advice proves 'bad' and you will not be grateful to them if it happens to be 'good' advice because people often rationalise these things to take credit for the good things and blame others for the bad. This way, it is better to listen and to offer options and logically list them with possible consequences. However, don't give instructions or take instructions. The most important life choices need to be owned and taken with full accountability. If mistakes are made, let them be your mistakes because they are the learning experiences that you need to face head-on and use that information to grow and change and evolve. If you listen to somebody else, you will legitimately (or not) be able to absolve yourself of responsibility of the consequences of your actions, which won't be good for you or those around you. In summary, conserve your energy and use it for things and people that are healthy, useful and worthy of it … and remove the rest, because they are not passive. They are actively destroying your life and using up energy that could be directed at achieving your goals and aims.

The Psychology of Auditions

I'm going to give two seemingly opposing pieces of advice and both are valid according to context. That might sound paradoxical but that's life.

I believe that some people should never audition for anything, because the process will restrict growth and life trajectory. However, I suspect that these people are a rarity. If I had to put an estimate on the number, I'd suggest that one in twenty people should not submit to an audition process because it will be restrictive, a waste of time, energy and not conducive to success. With that said I suggest that 95% of people, if they feel the need to audition should do so and do so as effectively and enthusiastically as possible.

Statistically speaking, with regards to auditions specifically, you will probably fail anyway, so what is there to lose? If you read the paragraph above and were triggered then I suggest that you are not the type of person who should even consider a route, other than the traditional i.e. auditioning, casting or submitting to someone else's decision. However, if you are the type of person who does not submit and feels that the process will be too demeaning, no matter what the benefit then, I have a great suggestion just for you!

Create projects for yourself and give yourself the starring role!

Not everybody is designed to do this, but it's easier nowadays than ever before. You have a platform with social media and the tools and technology readily available (to even film a movie if you want to!) to do so and although I can't offer any scientific data to back this up, only gut feeling from experience. If you are the type of person with the drive to create a project and push to its conclusion, then you will probably be able to push with a much higher probability of success than a simple audition where nearly every factor and variable to determine your success is out of your hands and control. I guarantee that you will learn more, grow and also enjoy the experience. You will at least enjoy the experience more than the 95% — 99.9% of people who are rejected.

The probability of audition success

I typed in to Google 'audition to booking ratio' and I am pleased to see that it correlates with my approximate observation of the industry, at best: 5% (or a one in twenty chance of audition success). **backstage.com** in a 2010 article entitled *Booking Ratios* by 'secret agent man' state:

"A booking ratio is exactly what it sounds like: two numbers that represent how many jobs you've booked compared to how many auditions you've had. So if your ratio is one out of 20, that means it took 20 auditions for you to land one job".

However, I would suggest that this is probably the average best case scenario because the author points out, in the same article:

"One of my most promising young clients has been out on something like 40 auditions and hasn't booked a single job".

In reality, people can audition much more than that and get 100% rejection. Cecilia Capuzzi Simon's *New York Times* April 2008 article "Tryouts for the Rest of Your Life" describes:

"all told, a record 1,200 students were auditioning for 16 spots in the fall acting class or 12 in the musical theatre program."

That's approximately closer to a 98% failure rate. I have seen successful people crushed psychologically because of repeated failed auditions. On the other hand, I have friends who got an audition and became some of the most famous people in the world. I suggest that you do take action that is conducive to your own mental well-being and corresponds with your own realistic chances of success. That means, that you may have an amazing record of success with auditioning and casting and maybe you enjoy it ... you should continue. However, I suggest that if this is not the case then you should invest in yourself and create your own projects because then at least you are in control of the outcome and ultimately you can control its success and impact in the world. However, there are relatively few people who will do the work required. Relatively few people who have the drive to travel down that road. Possibly less than 5%, which means that it's probably the same success rate as auditioning anyway, with the exception that you are almost 100% in control of whether you succeed or not, compared to almost 0% control when somebody else is making the decisions. With that said, only you know what is the best route for you. Here are some audition tips to increase your chances and also improve your psychological well-being before, during and after an audition.

Beware!

An audition is not a natural healthy environment. It can leave you feeling drained, feeling dehumanised and often rejected. Statistically, you will almost certainly be rejected with very little feedback. Although this is normal in the entertainment industry, this is not a normal in any other realm of life. It is completely reasonable to be upset by this or have a negative psychological reaction. However, it's best to know this in advance and take remedial action. There are obviously different types of auditions depending on your craft. Here are some quick general tips and pointers.

Audition tips and advice

— Get an agent! This will make your life easier and increase your chances of success.

— Read the audition instructions carefully in advance and follow them carefully.

— Good preparation is key.

— Always bring an up to date photo/picture and CV/resume.

— Always be professional and don't make excuses under any circumstances.

— Be consistent and resilient. If you choose to audition, go all the way and all in!

— Remember that your first impression is key. Walk in with confidence, good posture and smile.

— Keep your energy up until you leave the building/area, not just the room. You might still might bump into somebody important on your way out!

— Dress appropriately and if this is not stated, dress smart casual.

— Pick material that is personally linked to you, something that you are passionate about.

— Psyche yourself up and make sure that you prepare your energy levels so that you are ready.

— Make eye contact and don't worry. This is meaningless in the grand scheme of the universe anyway!

— Once it's over, let it go and refocus on the next one. Don't think about it again unless to analyse and actively work on improving your technique.

Expertise, Knowledge, Intensity, Respect

I am a strong believer in the idea that expertise and knowledge through intensity, equal respect. Respect translates to power and influence in your field of expertise. I also suggest that becoming an 'expert' in almost anything in the world focuses your mind and sharpens it so that you can then relate it to nearly all other life goals. I believe that it's about intensity. To become an expert in any subject or field you will need to utilise intense energy. This is needed to research, to absorb and to put the necessary energy in to require the experience to become an expert. That energy and subsequent experience will become useful and remains with you and will often translate into other areas of your life. In addition to this, your life will become easier because eventually if you become an expert in your field:

1. Clients will actually seek you out for your expertise and advice.

2. You will become respected in your field and respected generally for being an expert in your field.

3. People trust experts.

4. Your advice can rarely be questioned if you are the expert.

5. You will get media attention, might be called as an expert witness or even be able to raise your prices because of the level of your expertise.

6. People will want to get to know you.

Practise makes perfect

We have all heard the proverb 'practise make perfect', which means that doing the same thing repeatedly makes it perfect. Well, that is true but it's also true that you must practise the right way. The best way to do this is to work on something that you already enjoy, are already good at, want to do and have a mentor to help guide you, if need be.

If you put the work in to become an expert in your desired field, I guarantee that that energy, expertise and ethics will 'bleed' into all areas of your life and help you succeed creatively, professionally and personally.

You Are Not Your Talent

Beethoven, for me, was probably the greatest composer of all time. His piano sonatas are incredible. In fact, they are beyond that for me (and millions of others around the world). However, Beethoven was not his compositions. He was not his piano or his playing of that piano. He was not his music. It was the 'original nature' at his core. Ludwig Van Beethoven was a human being with incredible ability that changed the world but that life-changing ability was only a manifestation of his talent. It was a side to him and his abilities. He certainly wasn't particularly happy and was even arrested and put in jail for being drunk and disorderly on more than one occasion.

So what is this thing that we have to identify our talent with who we are? If we locked Beethoven in a room with just a piano from birth to death, do you really think he would have been happy and fulfilling his true meaning on this earth? To just compose music? This would be a tragedy. He himself longed for love and peace in his life, as do most of the great composers and artists. A certain disgraced pop musician often talked about being his true self on the stage and said that he could 'live and sleep' on stage. Have you ever heard anything so narcissistic in your life before? Look what happened to him… it's a cautionary tale of self-mutilation, self-loathing and child abuse. So if you desire to be 'one' with your talent and identify so profoundly with it, be aware that you may pay the price in the areas that really matter in your life. Even if you do so, 'real life' will catch up to you in the end and you won't have fulfilling relationships, love or equilibrium because that energy will have been focussed on your creative outlet.

So while your talent is a part of you, if you identify yourself as your talent it will soon become your prison. That kind of self-imposed bondage is absolutely the antithesis of artistic and creative expression, which should always be free and joyful.

It's important to realise that your talent is an ability you have, which is one of many abilities you have but it is not who you are at root. This is basic stuff and it's been propagated since the dawn of time. Even Gautama Buddha said that 'The root of suffering is attachment'. Another really important thing to remember is that if Beethoven's hands were chopped off in an accident, then his piano playing days would have ended that very moment. He was such a genius that he could have continued to compose, like he did when he was deaf but if he would have been so strongly identified with his piano playing and then have lost the physiological ability to actually play, then that would essentially be the end of his existence, certainly his psychological well-being and possibly even his life. Similarly, if an athlete dedicates their whole life and strongly intertwines their identity with their sporting ability, then at the first sign of physical incapability their personality would inevitably also unravel. It is certainly possible to achieve, live healthily and realise that your talent is a manifestation of your abilities but not the 'be all and end all'. Even if you believe this to be the case, life will show you otherwise at some point along the way. This means that not only is it unhealthy to identify with your talents, but it is futile. Ironically, when you accept this your artistic and creative energy will be free to really express itself and make an impact on the world, without your own imposed fears and psychological restrictions. Creative and artistic energy needs to be free to flow to its maximum potential.

A Star in the Middle of Nowhere?

If you have all the trappings of success and all of the context that that brings what happens when you are removed from that and put in a different environment? Can you still function with your full talent and ability? How do you even know that your abilities are real and intrinsic to who you are and not linked to luck, your location or the people around you?

So we remove the most talented dancer who has dedicated their whole life to dance and based their full identity on that talent. They live off the audience and the energy of being in that world. What happens when we remove the audience and they are placed in a different environment alone? We would potentially have a full collapse and breakdown.

However, the irony is that this scenario is not that unlikely. No human being can control elements that cannot be controlled. It doesn't matter how powerful you are, the world can change in the blink of an eye. Everything can be lost, in the blink of an eye, including your life. It's important to remember this because it helps us focus on what's important and actually live and experience, the moment. It might be a good idea for the artist to spend time alone to really analyse who they are, what they want and the level of their true abilities and potential so that it is powerful, strong and understood regardless of environment. That is true talent and power.

Motivation and Drive

What motivates you to perform; or create? This is such a pertinent question because it's essentially the foundation of what you do and will direct your artistic endeavours and in actual fact, your whole life. At the very least, this should ideally be conscious, rather than unconscious. Consequently, the question of whether your drives are an actual choice or compulsion is very important. Could your drive to succeed in any sphere of the arts or sports actually be a way of solving unresolved childhood or psychological issues? Could you be attempting to resolve them directly by performing or creating? Are you addicted to that process and could you let it go if you chose to?

It's important to really understand your motivations and the root cause of your drives because they may well not be positive for you. In other words, you might feel resolution by performing but in actual fact realise, later, that it didn't solve your issues and that you were actually running away from fears or from root issues in your life. Many pop stars have talked about becoming a musician to get girls. This is absolutely the case and not just a flippant remark. It's often as simple as this when we look at our true motivations. I would suggest that no matter what your true motivations are… let them be conscious and at the very least, understand them.

Once you've identified your drives … are you doing it right?

'Never give up' is a popular saying but it's crazy if you think about it. If you are doing things correctly and the way they need to be done to work and conducive to success, then continue. However, if things are not working then you should at the very least, give up on what you are doing and change course or change your actions and behaviours. If you have tried this multiple times for an amount of time (that only you can determine) and still a 'failure', then logic alone will tell you that it's not for you and that you should give up and try something else. Or a different way of putting it is to give up doing something the wrong way and start doing it the right way. Things can only work if you are doing them the right way. It's important to be honest with yourself and also to accept your own limitations and that things are not in your control. Not everything will happen the way you want them to happen… and that is fine. That is what makes life magical! The most important thing is that you ask *yourself* the question and don't listen to other people's opinions on what *you* should be doing because they don't know what your inner drives and motivations are. You owe it to yourself to know as this will help you succeed and live your life to its maximum and achieve your potentiality in a healthy way.

How do you know when I should change the course or give up?

Only you know the answer to this question. Writer Anthony Cerullo, in his article 'Why Science Says It's Okay to Give Up on Your Music Career Goals' from the sonicbids blog, makes a great point:

"One quick and easy way to judge this is with stress. If you're feeling so stressed about a particular goal that it has a negative effect on your life, then perhaps it's time to drop it. Goals are supposed to be challenging, but you shouldn't need sleeping pills to

fall asleep or be in a state of depression just to achieve them."

I agree with Anthony Cerullo completely.

Never give up… the real deal

There are some people, who do things the right way and have the drive and ability to succeed at their given task or artistic goal. As long as they are fulfilled and happy then they should never give up. It's as simple as that because it is that individual who will certainly succeed. Whether you are that person or not is a determination that only you can make. Either way, if you are right or wrong, it probably won't have any impact on the probability of success anyway, so it's important that you be honest with yourself so that you can put your energy and life force into something that will actually fulfil you and works for you.

The Next Project

'On to the Next One' is a song by the American hip rapper Jay-Z, from his album *The Blueprint 3* on his Roc Nation label. The song features rapper and producer Swizz Beatz. I can't pretend to be the biggest hip hop fan because I tend to enjoy classical music, however, I enjoy all types of music… especially music which is very good and Jay-Z has some great songs. I remember being very impressed by the music video to 'On to the Next One' but the song itself is very interesting and has Jay-Z rapping a mantra-like phrase 'on to the next one' repeatedly.

I can tell you that this is a very conducive mantra to success. It's simple, don't focus on your past projects … focus on your next one! This keeps you motivated and driven in the right direction. I almost never look back at my projects or even like to have them within my line of site. I intentionally hide my books from view, remove my dance DVDs and projects and put them away and only feature the current project that I am working on anywhere around me or in my environment. This will often be in the form of a computer desktop background.

One thing I do not do is celebrate past achievements because I put all of my energy into the next project. I think this is a wise thing to do. I do not mean that you shouldn't celebrate your achievements, because if you feel that you need to do so then that is great! I personally don't. I cringe a little bit when people congratulate me, for example after I have finished a book. However, I have allowed myself a small celebration when I reach the eight authored books threshold, which is my next one. I also allow myself to have a day off when I complete a major project. If I complete a major show or performance then I allow myself more time to physically recuperate though. However, my perspective is always to focus and move on to the next project.

A great lesson from film directors Francis Ford Coppola and George Lucas

Renowned film directors, Francis Ford Coppola (*The Godfather*) and George Lucas (*Star Wars*) had a great way of living on the edge and that entailed reinvesting their profits 'on to the next one'. This is also a great way to keep motivated when you are a high achiever. You've all probably heard the phrase 'eye of the tiger'. That was what Rocky Balboa had in *Rocky*, however it was suggested that his wealth and success had made him lose it. To get it back he went back into the trenches and almost started from scratch. The interesting thing is that to succeed you often feel like you have to have something to lose, as well. If it was easy then you probably wouldn't be motivated to achieve it anyway and put the work in required to attain your goal. So, Francis Ford Coppola and George Lucas knew how to grow and expand their empires by reinvesting their massive profits and success and directing that into the next project … with actual risk. This means that they certainly did not rest on their laurels but continued with the drive to expand and succeed. It paid off … in a massive way.

In a Forbes interview (31st December 2015), Adam Ozimek said that George Lucas "as a film maker made money in spite of himself, and he didn't care if his movies were a hit or not". I absolutely love this because this is one of the reasons he will go down as one of the greatest creative geniuses of all time. He also became the wealthiest film maker to date and certainly one of the most successful. Mike Fleming Jr, in a **deadline.com** interview (December 18, 2015) described Lucas's strategy:

"Behind many a classic Hollywood film franchise is a story of someone who gambled and won, and someone else who lost. The most extreme example of that is Star Wars. Depending on which side of the table you were on 40 years ago, the negotiations on those original pictures resulted in the greatest, or worst, deal in Hollywood history as George Lucas ended up with both the sequel and later the merchandising rights."

Fleming also interviewed George Lucas's former *Star Wars* lawyer, Tom Pollock, who answered a question as to why he made so little money from the first movie, "$150,000":

"The point was, at that point I was a lawyer doing what my client wanted. And what my client wanted wasn't the money, it was the ability to get the movie made."

In 2012 Disney acquired his company Lucasfilm for $4.05 billion. Proving that sometimes it does pay to create and stick to your own vision, regardless of the potential risk of financial losses because doing so can pay off in a much bigger way and be much more rewarding for you.

The Godfather and being an 'outsider'

Francis Ford Coppola is a creative genius and it would be an insult to describe him as only *The Godfather* masterpiece creator because he has created so many masterpieces! In a *New York Times* article (July 24th 1988), 'Francis Ford Coppola: Promises to Keep' by Robert Lindsey, he was described:

"Once part of the Hollywood establishment, he broke ranks to create his own studio but failed. Now, approaching 50, he is an outsider at once angry with industry moguls who stifle "creative people" and unsure of himself in the world they dominate."

This has always been the geniuses' way. He lived on the edge and reinvested to create even bigger projects. He took the risk and won. He was an outsider focussed on his mission, regardless of Hollywood. He is a very good example to look at, for any creative person, who is separate from his creative work; I am talking about his manner of working and getting projects done. This is such a great way for a high achiever to keep motivated. Just like in the 1973 science fiction film, *Westworld*, written by Michael Crichton and later the 2016 series produced by HBO series, people need to feel the exhilaration of fear and jeopardy to really enjoy the experience. It also pushes people to succeed because it gives the impression of having no choice but to succeed!

Financial management and the road to destruction in the entertainment industry

Even though the examples above turned massive risks into big financial successes, it's important to keep perspective and look at the full picture. The entertainment industry is littered with artists who worked their whole lives and died penniless, bankrupted or with nothing. It was reported that the now disgraced Michael Jackson was over $400,000,000 in debt when he died. *Business Insider's* Matthew Michaels reported, in May 2018 that, "Heavyweight champion Mike Tyson earned $300 million over his career but he was knocked down with a $23 million debt in 2003. He declared bankruptcy, returned to jail before he again reached financial stability". Rapper MC Hammer of 'Can't Touch This' fame had "$30 million in the bank" and later "declared bankruptcy in 1996 while he was $13 million in debt", reports Michaels, in the same article. There are many examples of talented artists mismanaging their finances and ending up with nothing.

5 financial tips for artists, creative people and musicians

1) Don't get into debt

If it's possible to not get into debt for a creative project absolutely don't. Be prepared to lose financially without it getting you into a financial hole as this will affect your future creative abilities to get things done to the best of your potential.

2) Get an accountant

Many artists find maths and accounting very boring and complicated. Find an accountant that you trust and stick with them. They will help you navigate the financial and tax world and also become a trusted advisor over time that can potentially save you from financial ruin.

3) Residual income and multiple streams of income

Create multiple streams of income if you can, especially residual income that generates money when you do 'nothing'. This is essentially not putting all of your eggs in one basket. You can read more about this in Think and Grow Rich *which was written in 1937 by Napoleon Hill and is available worldwide.*

4) Save your money

This is a simple one but often the hardest one to do. You can save a certain specific percentage of your money by way of routine or you can do it any way you wish…. Just save an amount of money and make sure it goes up and not down.

5) Don't live beyond your means

If you can master this, then you will be totally fine and very successful without exception.

Don't Look Up, Don't Look Down

Never look up to anybody and never look down on anybody. It's as simple as that. If you do so, you are at the very least, psychologically elevating yourself or you are demeaning yourself. The reason is simple: you are not below anybody and you are not above anybody. So it's at the very least unnecessary but also unhelpful for you. Ironically, I heard somebody very interesting say something which I agreed with many years ago. He is a man that is loved by many and hated by many … but on this point, he was 100% correct. Before Donald Trump was President of the United States he was asked in an interview, "Who do you look up to?" and he replied, "I don't look up to anybody. There are people that I respect." Love him or hate him; that was a very intelligent answer.

It's not only unhelpful to look up to people but it's also unwise because things change when new information is revealed. For example, so many pop stars that many people have looked up to end up disgraced after years of drug use. All-powerful dictators once loved and worshipped, just days later, dead in a jail cell or worse. Just look at what happened to Nicolae Ceaușescu and his wife, Elena Ceaușescu, in Romania. Masterpieces in the art world worth millions, used as collateral, investments and to boost reputation, reduced to worthless when revealed to be faked. Unless you know everything about a person, which is impossible, it's best you see them for what they are – just a human being, with flaws and abilities. Not above you and certainly not below you.

It might be an idea to instead be inspired by nature or a philosophy or a way of thinking or an attitude – these things can be worthy of admiration. Although, even these powerful ideas are not infallible. So, what do we have left? Well, we have things the way they are. There is no need to characterise anything or anyone at all and that includes yourself. Those characterisations are often barriers and walls of mental restriction. They restrict you and restrict you seeing things as they really are. That clarity of vision is what will help you succeed, express yourself to the best of your abilities and fully experience life around you. You don't need to be inspired anyway! You have all of the abilities that you need to succeed inside of you right now at this very moment. Sometimes you just need to be reminded of that… I am reminding you now.

Part 2

Maintaining the Creative Mind

Practical Advice and Techniques

The Traffic Light System

I have created a practical system to help sort out the "good" and "bad" people in your life and to make an objective determination as to their "category" of good or bad or somewhere in between. It's something that most people don't think about. Are the people I am surrounded by actually positive for me?

The system is simply a device that you can use to really think about the people in your life and look at whether they are actually a positive or a negative force, and what to do about it once you have come to a decision.

This is not an easy thing to do, potentially but I have created a technique which, in my opinion, goes a little way in circumventing possible cognitive dissonance and denial, which would obviously be a potential concern when addressing any such issue honestly. When looking at potentially sensitive circumstances, which may result in emotional pain, shock or trauma, many people will actually often deny a problem, in an individual or otherwise, exists, with an inability to accept reality. Could this be naivety or another reason?

Discernment challenges and potential naivety when looking at the people in your life?

We want to firstly:

1) Identify the problem
2) Identify its effects
3) Deal with the problem at the root and if possible remove the cause completely

The specific issue that I wanted to deal with head-on was the 'potential discernment and potential naivety' issue and its effects when honestly looking at the people in your life, past, present and future. First things first…

I **thought** about the potential problem.

This is a good start … but a terrible finish. I learned very quickly that you must write these things down in order to process them and identify them as a potential problem. Since the problem is concealed so we need to **convince ourselves** it exists with clear EVIDENCE.

Possible discernment challenges and its effects in regards to looking at our interactions

*1) I conceived a technique to write down the problem (possible discernment challenges and its effects) and a way to clearly see the issue on paper, **physically**.*
*2) I collated the data, **physically**.*
3) I applied the conclusions from the data directly and enthusiastically.
4) I measured the results.

The system I devised to identify possible discernment and naivety challenges and its effects on people is called, The Traffic Light System.

The Traffic Light System STEP 1:

Be in a Calm State – in a Peaceful Place

When you are in a calm state, find a peaceful quiet place to go and sit down. If possible avoid food or caffeine in the two hours prior. You want to be a relaxed as possible with a clear mind as possible.

You don't want to be disturbed for at least a couple of hours and you want to do this on a day when you can relax afterwards.

Pen and Paper

You will need pen and paper. If you *really* don't want to, you can use a word processor but ensure you create a clearly marked folder 'The Traffic Light System' and place that folder on your desktop in a clear corner of the screen. You want this to be treated with respect because this is important and it's YOUR life. Don't just save files and have them all over your computer. Everything neatly in one folder and respectfully positioned IF you're not going to use a classic pen and paper. I strongly urge you to do *that* first, and then later resubmit the information you are going to write down into a computer. There is benefit in the physical action of writing.

Create a List

Think about your life and the people in it. Think about those people. Your friends, your family, your colleagues, your relationships, your acquaintances … think about them. Think about their names. Think about their faces. Think about their physicality. Now write them down in a list. Literally a long list of names. Start the list with people in your immediate life right now. Somebody nearby physically. Then maybe your mother and father. Then maybe your boyfriend or girlfriend. If you haven't got a boyfriend or girlfriend, then you can write down an ex-partner. If you haven't got an ex-partner write down somebody that you really liked. Write down their name and think about that. Think about their look... you want to SEE them in your mind. Write down your best friend and then write down all of your best friends in your life. The list should be getting pretty lengthy now. However, it won't be unmanageable.

So now you have a list which will include:

Your partner and all of your ex partners
Your best friend and all of your ex best friends
Your family
Your work colleagues
Your acquaintances
Your enemies
Key people in your life
Your associates

You can add anybody else you interact with or have interacted with in any kind of meaningful way… within the last ten to twenty years. If you want to go back fifty years, do that. If you need to ask whether somebody specifically merits addition to the list, that means that they should be added to the list. If in doubt, add them. If the list is long, that's fine.

The List

You should now have a very random list of people in and from your life. It might be long, it might be short but ultimately this list is a list of your personal links, bonds and associates. In a way, it's a historical document, but it's *your* history. Did you notice that you might have felt a range of emotions when you visualised their names and physicality? Before we move onto the next step, have a look at your list and add any names that you may have forgotten. Those emotions and feelings are very important so don't worry about feeling too happy or upset or emotional about them, we'll deal with that in a moment.

The Traffic Light System STEP 2:

Put Your List Aside

If you wish, you can do this on a separate day to Step 1, however, it's up to you. You will have created a long list of people you like and people you dislike. People you love and people you hate. Put it aside now. If it's possible, put aside your feelings and emotions because we will address those shortly but for now, we have another task to do.

Get Your Pen and Paper

Using pen and paper copy these questions down (make sure it's a separate sheet of paper):

Question 1: How do I feel around this person *emotionally?* Good or bad?

Question 2: Do I feel good about *myself* around this person?

Question 3: Do I truly *like* this person?

Question 4: Do I characterise this person as a nice person?

Question 5: Does this person scare me?

Question 6: Does this person make me feel uncomfortable?

Question 7: Do I feel healthy around this person?

Question 8: Do I feel healthy *after* being around this person?

Question 9: Do I have a headache when I associate with this person?

Question 10: Do I feel like I can be my true self around this person?

Question 11: Do I feel good enough around this person?

Question 12: Do I feel valued *around* this person?

Question 13: Does this person uplift me?

Question 14: Do I characterise this person as 'negative' or 'toxic'?

Question 15: Do I feel comfortable being vulnerable around this person?

Question 16: Is this person a criminal or involved with drugs or illegal activity?

Question 17: Is this person a good influence or a bad influence?

Question 18: Do you like being around this person?

Question 19: Does this person 'uplift' you?

Question 20: Does this person 'bring you down'?

Question 21: Do you feel the need to filter what you say around this person?

Question 22: Do you respect this person as a human being?

Question 22: Do you trust this person 100%?

Question 23: Do you consider this person 'moral'?

Create a Folder on your Desktop Computer

You should now have a handwritten list of the above questions on a piece of paper and separate to that you should have a list of names. The next step is to create a folder on your computer (password protect this if need be) and label it The Traffic Light System. Within that folder create four separate documents labelled as follows:

1) Black
2) Red
3) Amber
4) Green

The Traffic Light System STEP 3:

You should open all four of the now titled documents on your computer and have your list on one side, in front of you and your questions on another side.

Then you should start with the **first** name on the list and ask each question of them, in your own mind. If you need to verbally speak it, DO IT!

However, specifically change the question from, say:

Question 21: Do you feel the need to filter what you say around this person?

To

Question 21: Do "I" (insert *your* name) feel the need to filter what you say around "**Mr or Mrs List**"? (insert *their* name)

You should add the **first** member of the list that we are looking at and replace "this person" or equivalent expression, to that specific person. You can do so in your mind or verbally. It is up to you.

What IS important that you actually ask the question.

What Will Start to Happen ... and the Rules

You will notice something very interesting happening. You will resist! You may fight your own mind. You may not even accept what you think, feel or even say! This is totally fine. This is part of it! In fact these questions are based on feelings and emotions and should be answered quickly and instinctively. If you hesitate and doubt an answer that immediately pops into your mind, then that could be your mind starting to rationalise and cognitive dissonance kicking in. This is also fine, but we have a rule and procedure for this.

The Rule

If in doubt, go *negative*.

If you have to think about the answer, for more than half a second, "Do I like this person?" then go negative. The questions are created to elicit an emotional unconscious response. We are not too interested in the reasoning and rationalisation behind said response. Now proceed through each question.

Physical Response and Facial Expression

You will probably have a physical response to your answers to these questions. Remember, it's irrelevant. We are just looking at some information and how that information manifests within you when triggered by a very simple mundane question.

Start With One Person Only

Make sure you start with one person only and then pause.

The Traffic Light System STEP 4:

Before we move on to the next step, let's take a look at the four folders that you have open on your desktop. Each folder has been assigned a colour and each colour has a very specific meaning. Take a look but don't worry about applying any meaning to them with regards to anyone specific just yet:

The Black Folder

– Threat to your life
– Threat to your well-being
– Threat to your mental well-being

— Psychopath, narcissist or Sociopath etc.
— A criminal perpetrator
— A scary person
— An enemy or somebody you feel that you hate

The Red Folder

— A negative influence
— A toxic person
— A horrible person
— Somebody that you actively dislike
— Somebody that you do not like (different from above)
— Somebody that you feel uncomfortable around
— Somebody you try to avoid and stay away from
— Somebody that is untrustworthy

The Amber Folder

— Somebody that you are slightly wary of
— Somebody that you like, but not all of the time
— Somebody that previously acted in a red manner but has changed drastically
— Somebody that you can't quite add to the Green folder
— Somebody that is usually nice but can have a horrible side when under pressure
— Somebody that has something off that you can't quite identify yet

– Somebody that you do not dislike and can see the good in them
– Somebody that you trust but not 100%

The Green Folder

– Somebody that you LOVE being around
– Somebody that you feel uplifted and energised being around
– Somebody that you love or really like
– Somebody that encourages you
– Somebody that you miss and wish you could spend more time with
– Somebody that you feel secure and safe with
– Somebody that you respect and are proud to know
– Somebody that you feel 100% safe around being 100% yourself

Person One on Your List

At this stage, you might know what to do already. In fact, you might want to get started already. DO IT! Person number one … ADD THEM TO THEIR FOLDER! Don't be shy and don't rationalise and excuse your initial thoughts and feelings. In fact the opposite: be STRONG. Your brain will automatically counter this by defending certain behaviour and rationalising and excusing. Remember, answer immediately and emotionally, based on your OWN understanding of the questions. There is no need to ask for clarification because this is a judgement based on your own understanding of the definition of those questions. However, be warned. It is irrelevant if you choose to cheat yourself and put somebody that you know is a black in the green folder because there will be real life consequences for that, so it's best that you do this honestly. Remember that this is 100% private and just for you, so it doesn't necessary have to have any impact on your life or behaviour if you don't want it to.

NEVER DISCLOSE THIS INFORMATION. IT IS 100% PRIVATE AND FOR YOU.

Start With the People Around You and Continue Through the List

It might be an idea to start with the most important people in your life, close to your orbit, so to speak, and then branch out through the list. However, it's totally up to you. Eventually, you will have four folders with a list of names in each. However, you may have no blacks. This is great! As long as you are being honest and truthful and you are correct, then that is wonderful. You may on the other hand, have no greens … don't worry… we will work on that too! The point is, is that you have the people in your life characterised according to clear motivations and behaviours now. Your feelings are based on how you really think *and* feel about the people around you. However, what should we do now? I will explain the next step! But before I do… at this stage you might encounter some issues.

Potential Issues and the Ideal Pyramid

At this stage you might actually experience shock and horror at the distribution of colours. I must say that I was. In fact, you can visualise it like this:

The Ideal Pyramid

Imagine a pyramid split into four coloured sections:

1) The Pyramidion
2) Upper middle section
3) Lower middle section
4) The foundation section

If you are imagining this in two dimensions, it would actually be an equilateral triangle but imagine that the Pyramidion is obviously the smallest section and this is coloured **black**. The second smallest section, just below this, the upper middle section is **red**. The lower middle section, the third largest section is **amber**. The final section, the foundation and the largest is the **green** section.

The Inverted Pyramid

Now imagine that the colours are switched. The Pyramidion is now green and the foundation is now black. The upper middle is amber and the lower middle section is now red. Now imagine that your pyramid (or equilateral triangle) is now *turned upside down*. That is what you call shocking and it should be a scary sight. If your distribution looks anything like the inverted pyramid, you need to address this immediately. In fact, you may very well notice that your distribution is closer to this than you would have initially thought! If it is then now is a good time to ask yourself why? Is this the first time you've noticed the people around you? Why is this? However, let's jump straight to remedial action. We can deal with those questions later!

Potentially Life-saving and Life-Changing Remedial Action

I strongly advise you to think about the results of your own thought experiment, the closer you look at the people you have around you in your life, and the people that you had around you in your life. It's important that there is a historical aspect to this so you can see how you evolve and if you learn lessons etc. If not, you can start learning from today and incorporate those lessons to changing certain behaviours or tendencies which may not be conjunctive to your wellbeing. I am not in a position to tell you what to do and I am a strong believer in that if you see the information in front of you, eventually it will seep into your life. You will do what you need to do. With that said. It's obvious and simple!

Spend more time with your GREEN lights and completely eradicate the BLACK lights from your life

A word about the black folder and other suggestions

I strongly suggest that you immediately and swiftly eradicate anybody from the black folder from your life. Do so swiftly, do so safely and do so with help and assistance if need be. They should be blocked out because if somebody is a threat to your life and well-being then that is a major problem. Seek help from a professional or law enforcement if you are scared to disconnect from anybody in your life. It goes without saying that the greens are where you want to be! Invest your energy, time, friendships and relationships in those. Be wary of the ambers but be open that they can change and people can change … however, they have their category for a reason, just remember that. Reds are a threat and also best out of your life. However, you might need to navigate a detachment in a more politically expedient way or even use your discernment with regards to work colleagues and situations which are difficult to remove yourself from. With these situations, you should consider the impact of proximity to said people and if need be, make a situational change … just do it, if you need so, in a controlled safe and reasonable way which works for your advantage.

An Example of Cognitive Dissonance

I knowingly mischaracterised one very textbook example of a red. This individual was clearly a red and I knew it straight away. However, for whatever reason another part of me didn't want to assign them to the folder I *knew* that they should be in. I rationalised many reasons. However, I made an illicit deal with *myself*. I turned a blind eye to it, after admitting to myself exactly what I was doing. This is fine… however, there were consequences and eventually the said individual was robustly placed in the red folder due to certain behaviours of said individual. Eventually, people will revert to type. The occupants of the red and black folders are THREATS. Threats need to be taken seriously and need to be seen as they are. Pretending that they are not there does not disable the threat or make it go away. I learned this lesson the hard way, but also took it very positively because it proved the point to myself practically. A red will act like a red, for example… and when they do, it's positive to know that you saw them for what they are accurately, even if you couldn't accept it, emotionally, straight away.

The Solution of Proximity

One of the best solutions is proximity. Creating distance between yourself and the problem or individual. If you can walk away, or move or just create an actual physical or psychological distance from the problem source, this is often the best solution. Utilise proximity regularly.

Looking at the Metadata

Metadata is defined as essentially, data about data. This is a GREAT way to look at things because it often removes the emotional element which can often confuse the situation. In a way, this is what The Traffic Light System is, it's an immediate look at the data, without too much emotional 'thinking'. However, you can take this deeper and can apply it to other areas of your life and interactions, especially if you are having problems in certain situations or with certain individuals. This is also a good technique to use in conjunction with The Traffic Light System. I will give you an example which relates to another book series I authored on Michael Jackson. I noticed that the professional media reviews were very positive and in actual fact, 100% positive. However, I noticed that certain associates critiqued and pointed out their negative viewpoints. There you have a very good example of a metadata data point. Professional critics were positive yet friends and associates point to their negative opinions. I applied a judgement on all perspectives of positive or negative but also, solicited or unsolicited, valid or invalid and then finally, accurate or useful (and also did I respect and implement any criticism).

I then compared and looked at the proportion in relation to each other and the metadata was brilliantly clear! In fact, if you remove the critique whether it be good **or** bad, then you can usually identify and predict the tone of the information without having to hear it, by looking at other factors, i.e. delivery, timing and context etc. That is INCREDIBLE if you think about it! You can predict what somebody will say, regardless by looking at a combination of behaviours and their usual traits. An example, 'friends and associates' that raised negative opinions or critique did these things **without fail,** I noted:

– They, without exception, started said conversation with the negative critique.
– They, without exception, pursued negative perspective exclusively with no positive feedback during said conversation as a counter balance.
– They, without exception, had an uncomfortable look on their face and displayed some degree of impoliteness.
– They, without exception, had not read the book they were critiquing (maximum one third of book).

– Were not professional critics or experts on said subject. In fact, were exclusively novices on said subject.
– Without exception, all feedback from these sources was adjudged objectively to be without merit and of no use.
– Their delivery, without exception, made me feel uncomfortable.
– Their advice and feedback, without exception was unsolicited.
– The timing was inappropriate, without exception. (i.e. I was in the middle of something, working, getting ready or preparing, or literally clothing myself…)

I realised that the **professional critics** were overwhelmingly **positive** yet associates and friends were overwhelmingly **negative**. Out of curiosity, I then looked at their traffic light colour and saw a correlation straight away.

The Reds and Blacks were the, without exceptions proponents of "negative criticism and points of view".

No green criticised at all!

That is a very important piece of information and

something you should bear in mind yourself ... always look at the **source and their motivations**.

Another part of looking at the metadata is looking at the **timing**. When did said individual choose to critique you, or point out something that would obviously upset you, or raise a negative point? Did they choose to do so at an inopportune time? I guarantee you, when you look at the timing you will see patterns with certain individuals.

Finally, when looking at the metadata the most important parameter is, "How do you feel?" Did said individual add value to your life or upset you (without any useful input) or just make you feel bad about yourself? If they are respectful, polite and offer constructive feedback and it is welcome, then that is acceptable. However, if you look at the metadata, you will soon learn that certain people project their nonsense on to you and they do so with the same predictable patterns and *modus operandi*. These people need to be removed or at the least within a reasonable proximity (away from you).

If you are asking questions about an individual or their motivations then that is enough to indicate a potential red flag about said individual. Their behaviour will not usually be a one off. It will probably be a noticeable pattern and trait in the person.

Meta Data in Summary

A good rule: "Did what the person said or do, which was not reasonable, upset you or make you angry or make you uncomfortable?" If it happens regularly then you should look closer at your association with this person and their metadata patterns. The fact that you are asking the question is the red flag but combined with the metadata matrix of timing, proportion (of conversation, i.e. was it 100% criticism?), the source, the value and was it solicited, you will start noticing the real feedback that is of value to you and consequently the **people** who are of value to you and disregarding those are not conjunctive to your well-being. It makes no difference whatsoever, what the subject of conversation is as the process is universal to anything which is important to you.

The Life Timeline

We've talked about looking at the metadata in others, however, that doesn't mean we ourselves can escape. This one is one which you can do once and it will help you give yourself a little bit of perspective and an insight into certain patterns or tendencies you may have, *over time.*

Things You Will Need:

1) A pile of A3 paper
2) A pencil and pen
3) A roll of sellotape

Step 1: Go to your calendar and work out how old you! You are going to create a timeline where 1 year of your life is measured with 10 cm. So, for example, if you are twenty years old, that would be 20 x 10cm in a horizontal line and a total of 200cm or 2 metres.

Step 2: Take your A3 paper and create a very long sheet, using the sellotape to secure the pieces together (on the back of the sheet, as you are going to write on the front).If you are twenty years old, you might want to make a sheet of 2 metres but also add another sheet so you have some space towards the left, and right, of the timeline.

Step 3: Now, take your pencil and plot out your life from your birthday and measure the distance until today. Each year should be marked with the date of that year. You will now see a timeline of your time on earth.

Step 4: You should now take your time and in a very relaxed way fill in the key moments of your life. You should label these points using a vertical line and a clear label. The key moments should include: major events and achievements, illness, relationships, work – essentially your highlights AND lowlights.

Step 5: You should now – on the horizontal line – build horizontal blocks and the distance and information within each block should relate to, say your relationship. If you had a partner for two years, then you should add that to the timeline. If you lived in a certain country or area, you should add that. You will now see overlapping boxes of information. It is very important that you put the low points (possible moments of say depression etc.). You can do this vertically which should give you more than enough space.

Step 6: Your income: go to birth and then draw a line from there until today. You need to create a vertical axis on the left with indicators from say 1 – 10. Then draw a line across the whole timeline indicating to, in your own opinion, what your financial situation was. If you were dead broke one year, then the line should be at zero. If you were rich for ten years, the line can go straight up and stay up for the horizontal distance of 1 metre on the sheet. The line itself will obviously go up and down but should not be disconnected at any point.

Step 7: You will now see the key points and moments in your life one gigantic timeline in front of you. You'll see where you have lived, your relationships, your high points and achievements, your low points, time of illness etc. It's important that you do this in pencil because you will start remembering things as you go and might have moments of clarity after you have already made notes.

The Final Step: The Happiness Line

On the left side you need to create a vertical line which is the 'happiness and content' measurement – say 20 cm vertical. Now you should start your line on the left, at birth, and then draw towards the right…a long long line! Look at all of the information and time on your own timeline and remember when you were happy… when you were happy the line goes up, when you were REALLY happy and content, it goes to the top! If you were down for a sustained period of time or a short period of time, the line should dip. Be honest with yourself and keep going until today. After a few days, take a look at your timeline. Do you notice any patterns of behaviour or anything interesting that you didn't realise about yourself?

Lessons Learned

This exercise alone can teach you more about yourself and tendencies and patterns in your life than any other. Just seeing the links and patterns and how they correspond with your happiness levels might even shock you. It will certainly be a revelation. You will also see how certain relationships and incidents impacted your well-being. You might note that you were always happy, when you were financially secure and felt down when you were poor. You might see that the happiest time in your life was when you had no money but was working on a piece of art for a year. The point is, for the first time look closely at your life. It will certainly inform you from now on and will have an incredible subconscious effect on you. It will also remind you that we are only on this earth for a limited period of time.

The Internal Furnace of Fulfilment

I wrote a book called *Living in a Bubble* about Asperger's and Autism Spectrum Disorder. I have noticed many similarities and parallels between the feelings and perspective of being on the spectrum and performers, artists and entertainers! In my experience, almost all artists identify as 'outsiders', as often 'lonely' or as 'different' (and I have noticed similarities in some abuse victims, also). Some of the techniques I created for people on the spectrum are certainly useful for any type of creative person that identifies with being an "outsider" or don't "fit in"… which is usually what being an artist is all about!

There is a technique which I know will help all of those people that find it difficult to connect, don't fit in or feel odd and isolated because of their personality, creativity, talents, perspective, interests or uniqueness and I've called it The internal furnace of fulfilment. It can help circumvent that "loneliness" and help you connect more but amplifying your uniqueness and creativity.

I suspect that most artists and creative people of all types (and especially those on the "spectrum"), if I say, 'living in my world' will know exactly what I'm talking about. They will understand the loneliness of living in that 'bubble' too.

Creative people can benefit by expanding that "bubble" and embracing their own uniqueness ... I will show you how!

I took a substantial amount of time thinking about this issue and how I would address it, in my own way, for myself. However, 'address' in actuality means, 'attempted address'. I visited Berlin, Germany and decided to use the opportunity to test some psychological devices and mental techniques to see if it could help with this 'living in your own world' or 'living in a bubble' issue.

The first couple of attempts didn't quite work, but then I worked out something which actually had a substantive impact. Before I explain and tell you all about it I want to tell you about a technique I use when I teach students in dance class because it relates to what we are talking about today.

Doing Something Physically Impossible

There are some dance moves that I teach that are physically and anatomically impossible to perform. This is because the human body cannot physiologically execute them. With that said I explain the process and then ask the students to attempt the impossible move and to *imagine* that it's happening. There has never been a single occasion where the physically impossible has been made possible … but something else has happened.

They came close!

The Challenge of Living in a Bubble

The one thing which I really focussed on was this idea of **feeling** like I was living in a bubble. How on earth can we solve that one? It's like you've been placed in a world with lots of people but you have an invisible bubble around you. You want to break out but you can't, as it's physically impossible. You see people walking past and people having their life experiences and you wish you could experience that too… but you can't because you **feel** like you live in your bubble.

How can you solve that? That's not an easy one to tackle for sure! It took me two years to come up with something that I'm willing to share with you, that I have tested, that I find works for me.

I felt like I made good progress with the 'Possible discernment and naivety challenges' and created a mechanism to try and solve that issue. So, I really considered the bubble issue in the same way. After two years of many types of mental techniques and psychophysical devices, on a really low day, it hit me. It was so obvious too.

How can you escape the inescapable?

Well, you don't, I told myself … you *EMBRACE THE BUBBLE,* that doesn't exist!

Embracing the Bubble and Living in Your Own World

The real pain comes from not necessarily living in a bubble but *feeling* excluded from what's outside of that non-existent bubble. However, this is 100%

psychological and emotional which means that the *solution* is probably also **psychological and emotional.**

There certainly is no bubble around you separating you from the world. It's a feeling only.
That knowledge alone is extremely empowering. Because it puts YOU back in control. You focus on what YOU can control and not what you can't and that alone is a very powerful psychological device in itself.

The irony is, I found that this route can, in actual fact, give you the *feeling* of breaking out of the bubble! It's like a back door route into the world. It takes a little work (but not much), it takes time (but not much) and the most important ingredient of all… it takes ENTHUSIASM and CONFIDENCE!

You will find that the world may well join YOU in your bubble because this will be attractive and infectious. However, the mental device is completely counter intuitive. I tested it in Prague, Czech Republic for about five days. I have called my psychological device, 'The internal furnace of fulfilment' and it's an internal validation system for you inside your bubble!

The Internal Furnace of Fulfilment

This metaphor is a psychological device designed to help refocus your perspective towards *internal fulfilment* rather than looking for and towards external validation and fulfilment, which helps towards feeling more comfortable within any perceived bubble and indirectly circumvents that same bubble, so that you feel even more connected and less excluded.

Here is the process and the rules and main points of The internal furnace of fulfilment:

1) You must have a passion that you can physically occupy your time and attention with, and put your energy into. This must be something that you enjoy and something which is not harmful to anybody or anything. If you don't have one, create one. As previously discussed in this book, it will probably be your passion and area of expertise. You then make a list relevant to your passion. That list should be impossible to achieve because it is so long. This is a very good way of shutting down excuses! For example, if you are an expert in World War Two history you may make a list that goes like this:

– Visit every WW2 museum in your city, then country, then continent, then the world
– Read every major WW2 book ever written
– Visit every WW2 historical site in your city, then country, then the world
– Discover things that have never been discovered before about WW2
– Write a book about your experiences and begin to teach about what you have learned
– Learn all about the aircraft of WW2. Work out a way to fly in a WW2 aircraft etc.

You get my point! The list is endless and it cuts off any excuses at source because this excludes the possibility of being bored or not having something to do. Now, in case your brain starts creating more excuses, like financial issues etc. then you can reorder your list to only include free activities first, until you have any required resources. Even then, you will have more than you can possibly achieve. If you need money, you will make money. If you can't work out a way to make money, then return to the free activities until there are no more to do, which is impossible, as you don't have enough decades on earth to even read all of the WW2 or History books in the library which you can borrow for free.

2) You decide in one moment that you will utilise The internal furnace of fulfilment. You mentally decide that from now on, your fulfilled comes from inside of you and that source is powered by you and only by you. The furnace is not a real furnace … it's a special one, because the heat (i.e. fulfilment, happiness, acceptance, validation) can only come from *your* internal furnace and secondly, the same heat generated by your furnace is **non-transferable**. This means that it is unlike real fire. It is completely invalid when it is outside of you and loses its energy. In the same way somebody can't give you their heat from their furnace. This means that it can only be sourced internally. This means:

– If somebody walks up to you and gives you £100,000,000 in cash, you accept in advance that this cannot give you any heat (i.e. fulfilment, happiness, acceptance, validation etc.).

– The most beautiful person on earth walks up to you and asks you on a date or to marry you, you accept in advance that this cannot give you any heat (i.e. fulfilment, happiness, acceptance, validation etc.).

– You are promoted to the CEO of the most valuable

company of all time and you accept in advance that this cannot give you any heat (i.e. fulfilment, happiness, acceptance, validation etc.).

– Anything nice, good or positive given to you, externally cannot give you any heat (i.e. fulfilment, happiness, acceptance, validation etc.).

3) You completely embrace your bubble and turn your lens inwards (to ultimately face outwards). This means that you, as extreme as this is going to sound, from now on expect nothing from anybody – regardless of the circumstance. In fact, you do not require acknowledgement or appreciation at all. No matter what you do! **You do because it is of intrinsic value and aligned with your passion and well-being or something you are required to do for the greater good.** The greater good is something which is a personal moral decision for you to decide on your own. If you determine that something is morally required or practically required, then do it. If not, don't. If you are selfish, you will remain selfish. If you are generous, you will remain generous. However, everything else which is outside of those exceptions is purely focussed on your passion or to that end. This means:

— You walk up to a stranger and help them pick up all of their dropped belongings. You do not expect a thanks. You do not expect even a look or the smallest amount acknowledgement. You may accept it but you do not expect it.

— You clean your best friend's house, from top to bottom. You do not expect a thanks. You do not expect even a look or the smallest acknowledgement. You may accept it but you do not expect it.

— You give away £100,000,000 to a charity. You do not expect thanks. You do not expect even a look or the smallest acknowledgement. You may accept it but you do not expect it.

— You engage in a conversation with somebody. You do not expect a reply. You do not expect even a look or the smallest amount of acknowledgement. You may accept it but you do not expect it.

Everything you do is focussed 100% on advancing your main life passion with the exception of actions which you determine are morally or practically required for the greater good or your own good, within your own personal moral spectrum. To repeat, the action is executed for its intrinsic value only, with zero expectation of acknowledgement or expectation that it will give you any 'warmth' or 'heat' except the heat generated internally from the 'power' of the intrinsic action and the heat from that. You do not feel the need to speak, communicate or receive anything from anyone, in particular.

How to Start a 'Metaphorical Furnace'

When you wake up in the morning, over the duration of this experiment, the first thing you should do is SMILE. The smile indicates a knowledge that your heat is generated internally… and that is GREAT news! Secondly, a physical kick start is required to start a real furnace so we too have a physical kick start to boost our *metaphorical* furnace. Here it is:

1) As soon as you open your eyes in the morning, you smile.

2) As soon as you stand up out of bed you tense your hands, chest and arms and at the same time, in three short bursts, expel air through your nose with FORCE. You should add three physical movements.

3) Simultaneously, with the three exhalations and forceful 'rocking' movements, you internally say "It's IN – SIDE – ME!" If you wish to say it out loud – DO IT!

Possible Side Effects and Results

If you feel sadness because you feel that you are excluded and live in your bubble then there is no loss in trying a mental technique to try and avoid feeling that way. The worst that can happen is that it doesn't work and that you feel sadness. With that said, I found that you may feel sadness for twenty-four to forty-eight hours when participating in a psychological device like this. However, it's my opinion that this is more to do with facing the issue directly. Once you see the positive effects and a short amount of time passes, this will pass and at the worst, even if it didn't work and it's all nonsense, you can resume your usual baseline of sadness. However, you will be shocked at the impact this technique can have… the positive results were actually shocking to me!

The results were absolutely counter intuitive … and I measured them!

Shocking Results

During the first half of my trip to Prague, Czech Republic I spoke with five people including the man at the taxi reception desk at the airport and very briefly with the taxi driver, somebody at the accommodation and two waiters. I had no meaningful human interactions than this, over four days. I decided that this was the time to activate my psychophysical device and did so on the fifth morning. I found that the first twenty-four hour or so, were very tough as I felt sadness, however, that soon passed. Then things started happening...

Waiter Number 1

During the first part of the trip I visited Prague Castle multiple times and I ate in the restaurant. I was served by two waiters. During the first part of the trip we spoke but only spoke about logistics. What I wanted to eat and sit etc. However, I returned mid-experiment and something very interesting happened. The waiter came up to me in a very friendly enthusiastic manner and greeted me. He asked me if I wanted the same as I had before. I was slightly surprised that he remembered what I wanted. It was a very nice experience and we got talking. We talked in detail about the differences between Prague in summer and Prague in winter. When we were talking, the next table got involved with the conversation.

Waiter Number 2

The routine went like this: I would walk around the castle and then go to the restaurant and eat. I would then walk around the castle and then go to the cafe on the side of the castle wall. After my restaurant experience, I walked to the cafe, which is outside. As I walked up the waiter, smiled and said, "Would you like your usual?" I smiled and said, "Yes, please!" He then added, "I've reserved your usual table and it's waiting for you." We both smiled as it was a small cafe, but he was right, that was the exact table. He explained that they were out of Coca Cola but had a new Schweppes Cola. He explained his thoughts and I tried the new drink. We talked and had a great time.

Return Taxi Journey

I had a very extensive conversation with the taxi driver on the return journey. At the end of the journey he said, "I wish I had more conversations like this one, here is my card, please call me the next time you come to Prague."

At the Airport and Beyond

I have a habit of going to the perfume section when I'm at the airport and testing out the perfumes. I just like the feminine smells. A perfume really does take you back and for me, it links me to, for example, friends or ex-girlfriends etc. I enthusiastically started to smell a perfume, which was the sister perfume of one that my ex-partner used to wear. It actually smelt really nice but not as nice as my ex-partner's version. I was mentally going through all of this in my mind and obviously visually doing so because a beautiful woman walked past and then looked at me, walked towards me and said, "Which one is that? It looks nice". I woke from my little internal dialogue with myself and said, "Yes", but that she should try the other one, which was better and explained why I wasn't smelling that one, and we both laughed. I then told her that I hope she enjoyed them, as I left her smelling them and off I went. Later as I sat waiting for the plane, she came and sat opposite me.
Before this I found myself in the middle of a wedding being held at the Prague Museum of

Technological and quite a few other random adventures. I calculated that I had had more than four times the number of the human interactions that the first part of the trip and they were really fun, joyous and interesting conversations! In addition, all of these interactions happened when I was in the middle of following my passion. For example, I was literally working through my Prague list of locations, museums, galleries and places I wanted to go, during which these things happened. During the second part of the trip I had such a great time with really meaningful and nice human interaction, which I enjoyed. As I write this, I return to Prague in five days … I enjoyed myself that much.

Enthusiasm and Extending Your Bubble to Include Others

If you walk into a bar, let's say and you are insecure and uncomfortable and feeling like you live in your bubble and order a drink. You, as well as not particularly enjoy the experience, will probably not have any enjoyable human interactions. However, the same you walks into a bar, which is linked in some way to your passion i.e., it's en route to a location, or is intrinsically linked historically or architecturally to your passion and you enjoy the interest in it for that alone, you will see things will happen!

At the very least you will enjoy the experience because it is aligned with your passion. For example, you walk into a special building with special architecture. You sit down and really take an interest in that architecture and the design of the room and the ergonomics of the table, the set design, the menus etc. Human beings are curious beings and are attracted to enthusiasm! So, when somebody sees YOU having a good time for real, SOMEBODY will want to be part of AUTHENTIC action. Just the same way, if you stand in a busy street and look up, people will look up too! Or stand and point, people will be curious.

At that time, you can explain your passion and at that moment, just for a moment, you have succeeded in extended your bubble to include them … in a bar! Even if nothing becomes of it, you've had a meaningful conversation, about something you enjoy in a location that is in some way linked to something you're passionate about. That in itself is a great thing and I can guarantee that if you keep doing this, eventually, your circumstances will change and your bubble will grow over time.

Not putting pressure on people or imposing your expectations on them is a VERY ATTRACTIVE THING. They will WANT to be around you if you make this a way of life because you will want nothing and provide enthusiasm, energy and value and be a living example of somebody that is brave enough to follow their passion. You will see… so few people have the courage to do it, that when you do it, you will be 'different' and if you already feel different, then you might as well embrace it and go all the way! In other words, embrace the bubble! That bubble can be your doorway to self-improvement, knowledge and living enthusiastically which can and probably will lead to, not you leaving the bubble but the world joining you inside.

Other Unexpected Benefits

– You will not tolerate disrespect, time wasters or nonsense any more

– Your value of yourself and self-respect levels increase

— You become more attractive

—You are filled with more enthusiasm

—Your contentment levels increase

— Your meaningful interactions increase

— Become closer to your life goal and passion

— You will become more generous and notice the "small" things more

And last but not least ... 'the 20%'

There is a proportion of people in this world that are real life heroes. I don't know if the percentage is 20% but I can tell you that these people are the people who have empathy and sensitivity and consideration. They will be the 'greens' on your list. Focus on those greens. Surround yourself with greens and invest in *them*.

Your Way Is the Only Right Way for You

You can find your own way… you can do it! In a way, nobody can give advice how to discover yourself and what works for you, except you. It's from within. You can evolve based on your own knowledge and experience. You are 100% in charge, you are the captain, YOU are the expert.

You won't get it in full, from this book, or any book because it is your duty and responsibility to create a process or routine or a plan that works for **you** in your life. On the other hand, you will get closer to the destination, regardless, because you can gain knowledge from any book, experience or human being in an apophatic sense. This means that if it doesn't work for *you*, then at least you *know* it doesn't work you. There is much value in even that. Focus on creating your *own* "guide book" for *yourself* through knowledge and experience.

Embracing New Things

1) Look to those you admire already

Try this trick! Think of the people you are a big fan of and respect. Maybe they are an artist, a musician, an actor, a scientist or a politician and find out what THEIR interests were. They probably have/had a variety of interests and talents that aren't publicised.

2) Force yourself to try something new

Make a list of your possible untapped talents and skills. You will be shocked because you probably, no… you *definitely* have talents in areas you haven't discovered yet!

3) Push yourself – don't let talent go to waste!

Embrace your 'weird' interests and make sure you don't fight against them! They are probably one of the biggest blessings of your life.

5) Express yourself in all the ways you can

Make sure that you express yourself in all the ways you wish and want to before you die. Most people don't and leave it until it's too late. Don't make that mistake – express yourself and your talents while you have the chance and make sure you enjoy the experience too. If you need help and assistance, ask a friend for advice and support. You can even say to a friend, "I need some encouragement with regards to this." Believe in yourself and others will believe in you. If they don't believe in you (or they do), it's not even relevant. They will believe after you have proven them wrong and respect you and admire you!

Maintaining your Talent and Staying Well

I told you at the beginning of the book that I was going to speak from personal experience. The next few paragraphs have the potential to transform your life. These things worked for me and they may work for you.

Fitness

Fitness and exercise affect my feeling of well-being and ability to interact with the world. My usual exercise is running. I don't count my dancing as exercise because that's also a mental activity; I am usually teaching as well as moving. With running, I can just run. I used to run up to ten miles per day but I found, after a time, that this took too much out of me. So now I can run an hour pretty easily and still feel fresh and strong throughout the day. Exercise produces endorphins which lift our mood.

I also see running as a social activity, even though I don't speak with anybody. I see people, I interact with them and this is a good thing because it reminds me that I am part of a wider society.

It goes without saying that any regular fitness activity will improve your self-confidence. If you incorporate a fitness routine, which you are comfortable with and enjoy, you will receive significant benefits to your outlook, mood, health and general well-being.

Sleep

When we're tired it doesn't help us interact with the world in a happy way. So it's important that you get enough sleep. How much sleep is a personal thing based upon your own body and your own activity. You want to sleep until you feel rested and then wake up. It's probably not a good thing to sleep for less than eight hours regularly but you should experiment and see what amount of rest helps you to feel best. For me, the way I am awoken is extremely important.

Get into a relaxed state prior to sleep – this might include not having a television or other screens on in the bedroom.

Food

We are what we eat and I have experimented for weeks with different diets and different foods and this is what I can report:

Sugar

Cutting sugar out will change your life. When I cut sugar out, I felt like a different person. My mood changed, as much as I became more patient and more tolerant. I also felt more energetic and more stable.

Processed Foods

I cut out processed foods and replaced them with, as best as I could, organic healthy real food. People commented how bright and vibrant I looked and I just felt more peaceful and that I could handle the world better. I can say that cutting all the processed stuff out completely transformed the way I felt for the better.

Milk and Meat

I found that I had to reduce my running from ten miles a day because my energy levels, without meat, were significantly lower until I replaced meat with fish. Cutting out the dairy also helped me feel better and fresher. You should experiment with what works for you. This may be without, meat or fish or milk, for example.

Incorporating All of the Above

When I incorporated all of the above, I often described it as life changing and feeling like a new human being. I felt that I was less emotional and less reactive. Experiment with what works for you. Whatever you consume, consume it consciously and take note of how you feel that day and the next day. If you need to keep a diary.

We've already looked at some possible options with regards to health, nutrition and fitness. Now we're going to look briefly at some other types of maintenance.

Meditation

I have meditated for many days consecutively. I can say with my hand on heart it has been life changing. However, before I tell you about the specific meditation I do, I would encourage you, if you wish to meditate, to find one that you are comfortable with and works for you. You can look online or in books. Another thing you can do is just sit peacefully. Turn off the electric gadgets and phones as well as the lights and just sit for a few moments and be peaceful. You will be surprised how many ways this benefits you.

Another brilliant way of relaxing the brain is to find a peaceful meditative piece of music, say, Erik Satie's relaxing 'Gymnopedies' and again, turn off all the lights and gadgets and just sit and listen. I currently mediate for around forty minutes each day, however, I'm going to tell you about an easier one that I did for many days.

It's called 'Isha Kriya' from an Indian Yogi called Sadhguru. He looks the part. If you want a meditation you want one from a guy that looks like this! You can do a short thirteen minutes per day and it's in three parts. You just sit on a chair and essentially repeat (internally) to yourself, "I am not the body … I am not even the mind", then you make a certain sound, then you sit peacefully. You can find out more yourself online through the Isha Foundation or find an alternative meditation that may work for you. If you can't find one then feel free to make one up!

Control Surroundings and Environment (Recuperate and Safe Spaces)

It's very important that you create a safe space in your life where you can recuperate and relax without being disturbed, for an amount of time which you feel recharges your batteries. I would suggest that you do whatever you need to do to make it the best it can be. Fully soundproof a space if you must; just make sure that you have a place in your life to retreat to when things get too much.
If you can remove yourself from noise and disturbance then this is the best way – by creating distance. Or move if an environment really doesn't work. Don't be afraid of change as this will improve the quality of your life.

Get up to date medical attention and any psychological help

Make sure that you see the doctor regularly and keep up to date with your check-ups and medication. Also, do not be afraid to ask for any kind of psychological help you may need.

Cultivate Human Real World Relationships

Remember that you must try as hard as you can to put time aside to cultivate real world friendships and relationships and invest in them. This is good for you but your friends can also help you in times of need.

How to Feel Great… have some Fun!

Okay, time for some child's play regarding the easiest way to feel great and stay in shape! It's really easy to change your outlook and feel great, and I'm going to let you into the secret. How to stay in shape, how to stay energised, how to just be well! Now, before I let you into the secret… I have to admit that I stole it, from probably the greatest actor ever: Marlon Brando. It's the secret weapon that I pull out when I'm feeling down or overworked.

As a choreographer and dance teacher, it's also my job to give advice on how much to dance and practice and exercise tips, But again, do you want to hear something that costs nothing and is so simple, that doesn't involve a fifteen-step plan and your hard earned cash, only a little determination? I always tell my students that the best way to stay healthy and keep fit is a) to dance and b) to run (although that's not the secret!). Trust me, I have heard every excuse conceivable in the book, why this is not possible. It's quite entertaining to hear the same excuses from so many different people! It's quite simple; although you might have to wake up forty-five minutes earlier in the morning. All you have to do is invest in a good quality pair of trainers (sneakers) and run daily… That's it! But of course, they would rather quote scientific theories on shock impact as if they're experts in Chondromalacia, Chronic exertional compartment syndrome, Great excuse syndrome as well as other knee disorders…Anything not to, in the words of Nike "Just do it!"

Anyway, I digress!

It's really simple and is also the perfect way to jump into dance and any physical activity, especially for absolute beginners. Although it is very simple, it's something that so many people are unable to do. The number one way to lose weight and get into dance and get your backside moving! The bad news is that you won't want to hear it. It's probably too simple for you to accept!

The Secret

Marlon Brando. The man. Marlon Brando had the most amazing ability to lose weight. I mean, seriously, he would go from being a very healthy lean looking movie star to a massively overweight man, and then back again, in very short periods of time…But how? He was once asked in an interview, "How do you lose weight so quickly?" Now, you'd be surprised at his answer. Did it involve an army of Hollywood trainers? No! Did it involve subscribing to nonsensical unhealthy scam diets? No! It was completely free… and very easy to do. He would close the curtains, close the doors, put on a great piece of music full blast… and just go crazy! Yes, just move to the music. No choreography, no nothing! He said that he just copied the Hula dancers that he watched, with all that movement. You are a human being, with natural rhythm…Why do you need to learn to go enjoy a great happy song? You don't. And I mean, go crazy… Just do whatever you feel like, manoeuvre like a crazy beast… Just lose control for once. Feel free to lose your inhibitions and be free! Hey, nobody's watching, so who gives a damn anyway!

Marlon Brando filmed and vacationed in Hawaii, and was inspired and impressed by the natural movements e.g. natural dance like the Samburu tribe dance, in Africa. Forget this nonsense that you have to learn how to do this, or learn how to do that or that you can only lose weight and keep fit and feel good with a yearly membership at the top gym, that you hardly attend anyway, repeating mechanical, totally unnatural, robotic movements in front of a flashing box. Which is a totally new phenomenon anyway. You tell me where the healthiest people in the world are. Not in the same locations as the countries with the most gyms, I bet!

As every philosopher has said, it's always a case of 'unlearning' rather than 'learning'. And one more thing, mentally, you will feel great afterwards too. For once, really do something spontaneous and give it a try! That is my personal feel-good keep fit advice: the technique that I employ when I'm feeling down. Now, as always, it might be too complicated for many people to do something so simple – but why not give it a try? It's the perfect place to start for a beginner and I guarantee that you'll feel great afterwards and really be in a better position to advance and learn, as well as keep in shape. My Top five personally recommended songs are:

1) 'Le Freak' by Chic
2) 'Venus' by Bananarama
3) 'I Will Survive' by Gloria Gaynor
4) 'Manic Monday' by the Bangles
5) 'Puttin' on the Ritz' performed by Fred Astaire

Good luck! Think about your mental ability to try new things and not disregard something that may indeed help you. That simple thing might be something that you could use to progress. Don't disregard anything just because it sounds too simple. Advancement in the physical really does start in your head.

Conclusion: Acquiescing

We've already determined that one day we will probably be old and grey and that we will probably ask ourselves some very interesting questions about the way in which we lived our lives. Did we let the world and the people around us determine the direction of OUR lives, dreams and goals? Or were we one of the few who did not acquiesce? Who did not compromise? Who had the courage and the sense to achieve whatever it was that we wanted to achieve that made us happy?

Unfortunately, the sad truth is that if any of us is one of those people, we are in a lonely minority. The majority will capitulate to societal pressure and the people around them. They will do it silently, without realising that they could have changed the situation at any time by speaking out. Some might have eventually realised that it didn't have to be that way…but it'll be too late by then. We only have one chance. To take what's ours, while we still can. If you are an artist, always remember that you have the power to change your environment and your life.

What can I say that you don't already know? You are the number one expert in your life. So I ask you: How will you conclude? I'm curious…

Hopefully with some kind of action that will bring your dreams into reality…

I wish you success!

Anthony

Source Notes

The Secret Teachings of All Ages by Manly P. Hall (Originally published: 1928) - Pythagoras

Dance Like the Stars by Anthony King (Originally published: 2007)

The Merchant of Venice by William Shakespeare (16th-century) - act 5, sc. 1, l. 54

"Most people are other people… their passions a quotation" - Oscar Wilde

"… society is our extended mind and body." - The Culture of Counter Culture (Alan Watts

CE Tuttle Company, 1998)

"Our doubts are traitors, And make us lose the good we oft might win, By fearing to attempt."

By William Shakespeare, "Measure for Measure" Act I Scene IV (16th-century)

"Accept nothing as true that is not self-evident"- René Descartes

The Seven Habits of Highly Effective Teens (1998) by Sean Covey:

"You better get secretarial work or get married." Emmeline Snively

"I would say that this does not belong to the art which I am in the habit of considering music."

A. Oulibicheff

"Who the hell wants to hear actors talk?" H. M. Warner

"The horse is here to stay but the automobile is only a novelty – a fad."

The president of the Michigan Savings Bank advising Henry Ford's lawyer not to invest in the Ford Motor Co. 1903.

"We don't like their sound, and guitar music is on the way out." Decca Records

"Television won't last because people will soon get tired of staring at a plywood box every night."

Darryl Zanuck

"… good enough for our transatlantic friends … but unworthy of the attention of practical or scientific men." British Parliamentary Committee

"Sure-fire rubbish." Lawrence Gilman, reviewing Porgy and Bess by George Gershwin in the New York Herald Tribune, 1935.

"If excessive smoking actually plays a role in the production of lung cancer, it seems to be a minor one." W.C. Heuper, National Cancer Institute, 1954.

"The singer (Mick Jagger) will have to go; the BBC won't like him." Eric Easton

"It will be gone by June." Variety magazine's thoughts on rock 'n' roll in 1955.

Sir Kenneth Robinson - Do schools kill creativity? https://www.ted.com/talks/ken_robinson_says_schools_kill_creativity?

The 7 Habits of Highly Effective People by Stephen Covey (1989)

https://en.wikipedia.org/wiki/Hern%C3%A1n_Cort%C3%A9s#Destroying_the_ships - Hernán Cortés (destroying the ships)

Think and Grow Rich by Napoleon Hill, 1937 (Page 23 and 24) 1937

https://www.britannica.com/event/Chicago-fire-of-1871

https://www.history.com/topics/19th-century/great-chicago-fire

My Wage, Jessie B. Rittenhouse

The Count of Monte Cristo by Alexandre Dumas (1844)

Massive Attack, Angel (YouTube Official)
https://www.youtube.com/watch?v=hbe3CQamF8k

Robinson737
https://www.youtube.com/channel/UCwqXV1DF-wbX2XfY8FwVPPw

https://massiveattack.ie/info/angel

Facing your Fears (a PERSPECTIVE NEUROSCIENCE article – Science 15 Jun 2018: Vol. 360, Issue 6394, pp. 1186-1187 DOI: 10.1126/science.aau0035)

By Paul W. Frankland and Sheena A. Josselyn in Science magazine

https://en.oxforddictionaries.com/definition/principle

"Michael Jackson Stans React to 'Leaving Neverland' with Bus Ads and Death Threats" By Jamie Lee Curtis Taete

Mar 1 2019, 5:24pm – Vice News:
https://www.vice.com/en_us/article/panm5y/michael-jackson-stans-react-to-leaving-neverland-with-bus-ads-and-death-threats

https://www.backstage.com/magazine/article/booking-ratios-1-58974/

backstage.com 2010 "Booking Ratios" by 'secret agent man'

Cecilia Capuzzi Simon's New York Times April 2008 article "Try-outs for the Rest of Your Life"

https://www.nytimes.com/2008/04/20/education/edlife/theater.html

'Why Science Says It's Okay to Give Up on Your Music Career Goals' By Anthony Cerullo from the sonicbids blog

http://blog.sonicbids.com/why-science-says-its-okay-to-give-up-on-your-music-career-goals

https://www.forbes.com/sites/modeledbehavior/2015/12/31/sorry-george-lucas-but-star-wars-proves-the-profit-motive-can-be-good-for-art/

Geroge Lucas, Forbes interview (31st December 2015), by Adam Ozimek

Mike Fleming Jr, in a deadline.com, interview Geroge lucas (December 18, 2015):

'Star Wars' Legacy II: An Architect Of Hollywood's Greatest Deal Recalls How George Lucas Won Sequel Rights

https://deadline.com/2015/12/star-wars-franchise-george-lucas-historic-rights-deal-tom-pollock-1201669419/

'Francis Ford Coppola: Promises to Keep' by Robert Lindsey, New York Times article (July 24th 1988)

https://www.nytimes.com/1988/07/24/magazine/francis-ford-coppola-promises-to-keep.html

Business Insider, by Matthew Michael reported (May 2018): https://www.businessinsider.my/rich-famous-celebrities-who-lost-all-their-money-2018-5/

The Traffic Light System and Maintaining the Creative Mind, Practical Advice and Techniques from "Living in a Bubble" by Anthony King (2019)

The Seven Habits of Highly Effective Teens (1998) by Sean Covey

Sadhguru Meditation: https://www.ishafoundation.org/Ishakriya

"Six timeless marketing blunders" by William L. Shanklin (1988 - Page 77)

"The Not Terribly Good Book of Heroic Failures" by Stephen Pile (2012)

Special Thanks

Dr Cho Cho Khin
Karsten, Hege, Kasper and Taran
Mohammed Nabulsi
Rolfe Klement (Creative Sunshine back cover photography)
Debz Hobbs-Wyatt
Aimee Coveney
Jason and Marina
Sammy Ewan
The "LN" Twitter group
Dr Lunich
Therese and Eivind
Faisal Abbas
Luke Long

About the Author

Anthony King is a choreographer who started teaching dance at the world-famous Pineapple Dance Studios, London in 2004 and has authored seven books on a variety of subjects, from Dance to Asperger's to Music history. He has taught stars from music, sport and film including Emma Watson, Miss World, Harry Potter, various members of royalty (European and Middle Eastern), Pink Floyd, Top of the Pops, The Jonathan Ross show, Richard and Judy Show, Britain's Got Talent, BBC's EastEnders, BBC's The Office, and the England football team. Choreographed fashion shows for Vidal Sassoon, Anthony has starred in and choreographed commercials for Sony PlayStation, Maverick Media, Warner Music and more. Anthony is the original choreographer of the west end musical, 'Thriller Live'. Anthony has held dance team building events and workshops for the world's biggest companies from Twitter to Google, HM

Treasury Department, Lego, Capgemini, Anglo American, PwC, Bonnier Publishing, King (creators of Candy Crush), City Sprint, Red Bull, Cisco Systems, TK Maxx, American Express, Proctor & Gamble, Metro Newspaper group, Rimmel London and many more. He has been interviewed on most of the world's national and International media including Sky News, BBC News, BBC Breakfast, Channel 4, Channel 5, ITV, ITV 2, CNN, ITN, BBC Radio 1, Capital FM, Choice FM, BBC Radio London and many more. His online lessons have been viewed over 35 million times as well as being featured on YouTube homepage on numerous occasions. His classes have been described by the The Sun newspaper as 'Hot!' 'Elle girl' magazine have featured his classes as the 'NEXT BIG THING' as well as "dynamic and charismatic" by the London Lite. The Financial Times of London has recommended and featured Anthony's classes and he has been featured as a contributing writer for magazines including 'MORE MAGAZINE' as 'Celebrity dance tutor'.

Anthony King's Online Consultations

If you'd like to contact Anthony personally with regards to personal online consultations for help, advice or just to talk about any subject from this book please email: info@anthony-king.com or see www.anthony-king.com for more details.

Also by the Author

Living in a Bubble: A Guide to being diagnosed with High Functioning Asperger's as an Adult

The Dance Book – (coming in 2019)

Michael Jackson Fact Check – Fact checking the Michael Jackson 'experts'

Michael Jackson and Classical Music

Anthony King's Guide to Michael Jackson's Dangerous Tour

Anthony King's Guide to Michael Jackson's HIStory Tour

Printed in Great Britain
by Amazon